BEER VS BITTERS

Big Stepper

Chase DuQuesnay EnQi ReaL

Amazon

CONTENTS

INTRODUCTION

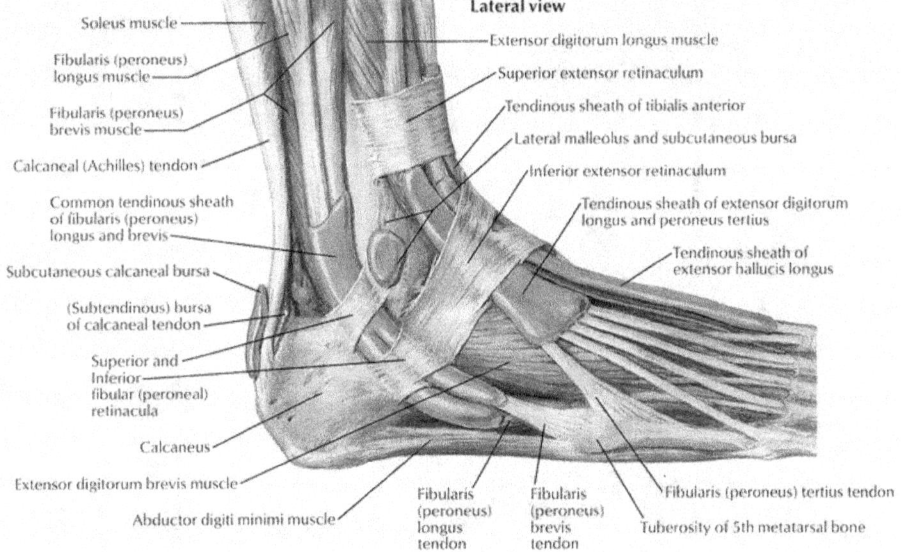

Tendon of flexor hallucis longus
Flexor hallucis brevis
Abductor hallucis (cut and retracted)
Tendon of flexor digitorum longus
Tendon of tibialis posterior
Quadratus plantae
Flexor digitorum brevis (cut)
Calcaneus
Tendons of flexor digitorum longus
Tendons of flexor digitorum brevis (cut)
Lumbricals
Abductor digiti minimi (cut)
Flexor digiti minimi brevis
Tendon of fibularis brevis
Tendon of fibularis longus
Abductor digiti minimi (cut)
(c) Plantar view, deep layer
Fibrous tendon sheaths
Flexor hallucis brevis
Abductor hallucis
Flexor digitorum brevis
Calcaneus
Lumbricals
Tendons of flexor digitorum brevis overlying tendons of flexor digitorum longus
Flexor digiti minimi brevis
Abductor digiti minimi
Plantar aponeurosis (cut)
(b) Plantar view, superficial layer

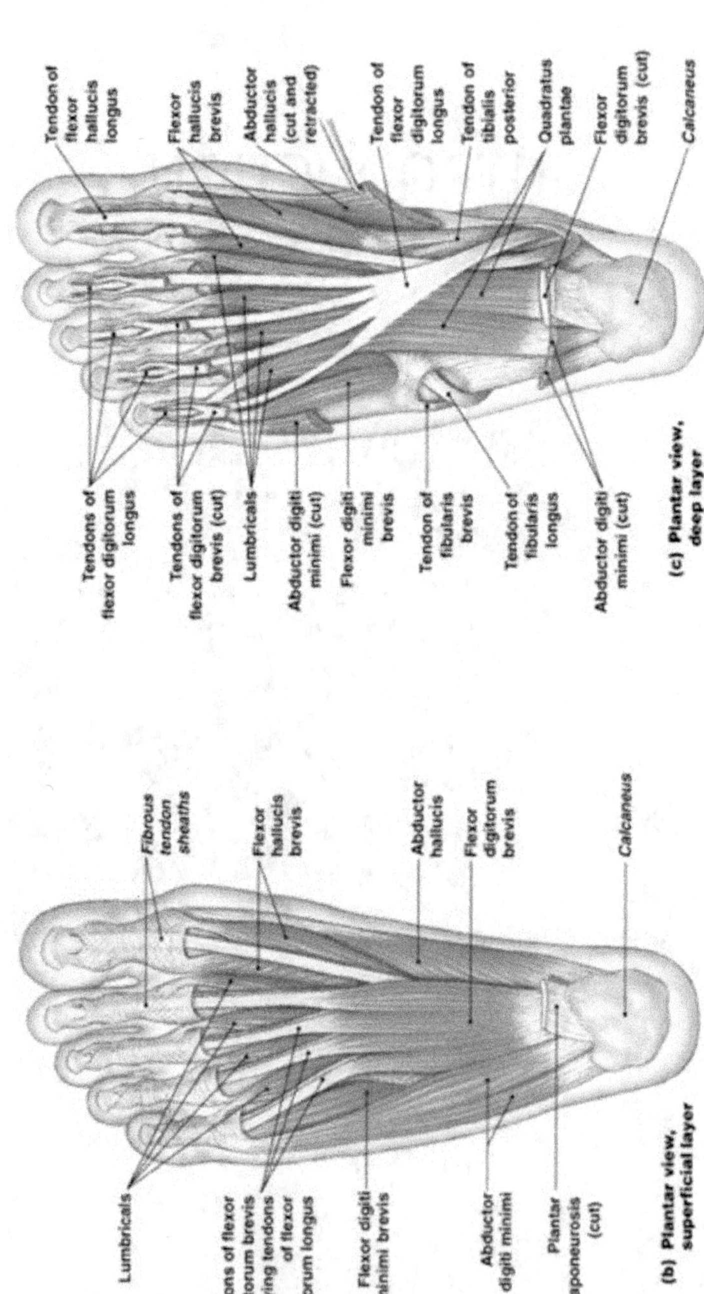

VI

FOREWORD

In Race Hustlers 5/Kemetic Science 1, the Movement book we discuss the Waveguide working through the spine, now as adults the hips, ribs, skull and sternum produce blood but the **spine** produces blood as well as recieved those signals. We are covering major major ground here!

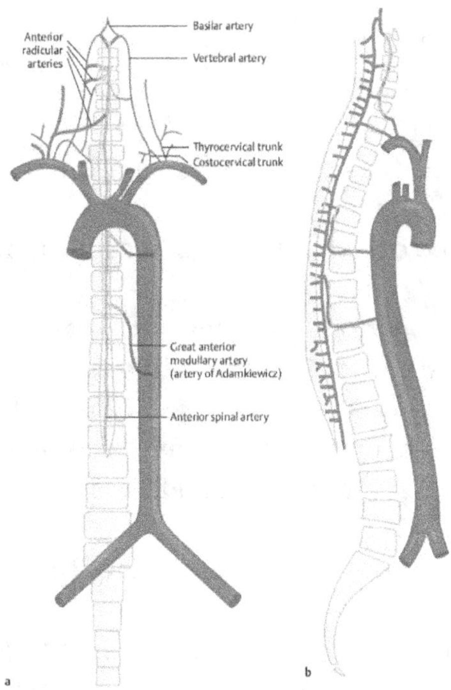

The blood is going from the spine or Djed directly into the Aorta!!!

In the Book of Two Ways, Re swallows the spine and spits out the day. We interpret that as a reference to the sun creating the waveguide and the waveguide speaking to our cells via the spine. The spine is seen as a substrate that is converted or metabolized into daylight.

In coffin text 577 & 1084 Osiris is called the Lord of Redness...

This bring the Ankh-Was-Djed into even more clear focus! The skeletal muscle we have discovered creates critical movement/ vibration the blood needs to maintain its structuring or spiraling. That perpetual movement is where the power is generated. Sugar crystalizing on the pigment and overall inhibiting pigment formation (inhibiting aromatic amino metabolism and destroying vitamin A), is the key to understanding how diabetes cripples the body.

Sugar coated blood does not have the proper spin.

Sugar coated blood does not carry oxygen and nutrients.

Sugar coated blood does not lead transport proteins properly.

Sugar coated blood does not have the same electromagnetic repulsion required to function in capillaries.

Sugar coated blood does not supply the skeletal muscle with enough energy, to create the ebb and flow of active muscle.

Sugar coated blood does not feed the rest of the body's cells.

Sugar coated blood primes the skeletal muscles with excess insulin receptors, prequisite for becoming cancerous, as a survival mechanism.

Sugar coated blood starves the body's cells while not absorbing oxygen at the same time, this low oxygen environment creates the need for fermentation especially with excess insulin receptors.

Cold hands and/or feet or feeling overall cold can be a warnning that the liver, brain, heart & skeletal muscle is not getting enough hormesis, so the countercurrent heat exchange is out like a bad radiator. The legs being the largest muscles need the most exercise and our lifestyle of sitting directly inhibits blood flow to the legs. Focusing our attention daily from the 19 vertebrae of the spine to the 19 muscles in the foot via exercise is beyond a good execrise, its just as crucial as breathing.

H2S maybe a polar haplotype or pheomelanin dominant protective mechanism where as eumelanin dominant or equatorial haplotypes produce high amounts of CO2. There also is potentially more fermentation via the type 2 fast twitch muscle.

Our research has pointed us to the heart and its 12 divisions being the throne of Osiris, the underworld being the world of your biochemistry, beer and bread must have had a diirect benefit to the heart! Kemetic Science is undefeated!

TRANSLATION

The shameful truth of ignorant Khemetic Scholarship, the Ankh has been identified as the womb of Isis and the Djed Pillar has been identified as the spine of Osiris, with the Was Scepter identified as Antelopes! How can that make sense in the context of Ankh-Was-Djed? Before we continue our mini-series inside our larger Kemetic Science series, we must show you a BLATANT EXAMPLE OF IGNORANCE!!! Within the following pages you will see some Original Text on the Was Scepter and you will see the translations of Antelopes vs Aorta in place of the Was Scepter. The challenge is simple, read them and see which one makes sense.

The gods, either male or female, carry the staff most often in conjunction with an anx sign (note fig. 1). anx is generally translated as "life,"13 while wAs may be translated into "do-minion," or "lordship,"14 suggesting that the gods are not only the possessors of sovereignty over the universe, but they carry eternal life with them. In this context, the staff became symbolically relevant and potent for funerary beliefs. Within Spell 1130 of the Coffin Texts, a deity who is called "Him whose names are secret" is quoted as saying "I possess life (anx), because I am its lord, and my staff (wAs) will not be taken away,"15 recalling this imagery of the gods carrying both the wAs scepter and anx sign together....
the wAs scepter and the anx sign also function as tools used during the "hourly vigil"17 to reanimate the corpse of Osiris after he is embalmed. In CT Spell 754, Osiris says to Horus "How happy are those who see, how content are those who hear, when Horus is seen ex- tending the wAs-staff to his father Osiris,"18 while in Book of the Dead Spell 146, Horus is quoted as saying "I am Horus,

the son of Osiris... I have brought life (anx) and dominion (wAs) to my father Osiris."......

570A: "This Pepi will sweep away with you (the imperishable gods) with a staff of authority (wAs) and an electrum staff (Dam) ...

BLOOD, ELECTRUM & OSIRIS ARE GREEN JUST A FYI!!! THE PERSIANS CALLED ELECTRUM, GREEN GOLD!!!

The gods, either male or female, carry the staff most often in conjunction with an anx sign (note fig. 1). anx is generally translated as "life,"13 while wAs may be translated into "antelopes," or "fantastic animals,"14 suggesting that the gods are not only the possessors of sovereignty over the universe, but they carry eternal life with them. In this context, the staff became symbolically relevant and potent for funerary beliefs. Within Spell 1130 of the Coffin Texts, a deity who is called "Him whose names are secret" is quoted as saying "I possess life, because I am its lord, and my (antelopes) will not be taken away,"15 recalling this imagery of the gods carrying both the antelopes scepter and anx sign together....

the antelopes and the anx sign also function as tools used during the "hourly vigil"17 to reanimate the corpse of Osiris after he is embalmed. In CT Spell 754, Osiris says to Horus "How happy are those who see, how content are those who hear, when Horus is seen ex- tending the antelopes to his father Osiris,"18 while in Book of the Dead Spell 146, Horus is quoted as saying "I am Horus, the son of Osiris... I have brought life (anx) and (antelopes) to my father Osiris."......

570A: "This Pepi will sweep away with you (the imperishable gods) with a staff of antelopes and an electrum staff (Dam)...

BLOOD, ELECTRUM & OSIRIS ARE GREEN JUST A FYI!!! THE SUN IS GREEN ALSO!!!

The gods, either male or female, carry the staff most often in conjunction with an anx sign (note fig. 1). anx is generally translated as "life,"13 while Aorta (or Blood) may be translated into "do-minion," or "lordship,"14 suggesting that the gods are not only the possessors of sovereignty over the universe, but they carry eternal life with them. In this context, the staff became symbolically relevant and potent for funerary beliefs. Within Spell 1130 of the Coffin Texts, a deity who is called "Him whose names are secret" is quoted as saying "I possess life, because I am its lord, and my Aorta (or Blood) will not be taken away,"15 recalling this imagery of the gods carrying both the Aorta (or Blood) and LIFE sign together....

the Aorta (or Blood) and the LIFE sign also function as tools used during the "hourly vigil"17 to reanimate the corpse of Osiris after he is embalmed. In CT Spell 754, Osiris says to Horus "How happy are those who see, how content are those who hear, when Horus is seen ex- tending the Aorta (or Blood) to his father Osiris,"18 while in Book of the Dead Spell 146, Horus is quoted as saying "I am Horus, the son of Osiris... I have brought life and the Aorta (or Blood) to my father Osiris.".....

570A: "This Pepi will sweep away with you (the imperishable gods) with a Aorta (or Blood) and an electrum staff (Dam)...

When translating you have to check your translation to make sure it makes sense. The question is now simple, does it make more sense that a womb and antelopes can resurrect Osiris (the spine) or that a womb and the aorta can resurrect Osiris (the spine)?

The Aorta as you will see from the IB book and the Was is the Aorta book (please read or reread those books), is the major tool of the Heart. The sidelock was associated with this science and many have distorted the historical narratives from these people.

OSIRIS, DIABETES & RESPIRATION

Anaerobic Respiration is almost the same as Aerobic Respiration regarding electrons moving through the electron transport chain. Different organisms have different final electron acceptors at the end of the electron transport chain.

Cells that live in low-oxygen environments rely on anaerobic respiration to break down fuels. Humans being the Master Cell Line have the super powers of all the simpler cell lines. The ability to produce energy from plain water, the ability to use oxygen and sugar or the ability to use sugar fermentation (glycolytic) for energy production. Pheomelanin Dominant people produce H_2S which has the unique smell of Sulfur to it. Equatorial Haplotypes don't have the abundant sulfur thiols present, this means a much higher output of CO_2! The reason for the big wide noses... Fermentation pathways are the same as glycolysis with some extra steps at the end. Yeast make alcohol this way, while in your muscles, they make lactic acid. This is very important regarding your health and the story of Osiris.

Your liver metabolizes 95% of the alcohol in your body, the rest goes out urine, sweating, breathing, saliva and feces. That means there is a small portion of alcohol that can be metabolized without notice.

Alcohol is oxidized to acetaldehyde then acetic acid then CO_2 & H_2O. Most people can metabolize half a ounce of alcohol a hour on average.

Drunk Without Drinking: A Case of Auto-Brewery Syndrome

Akhavan, Bobak J. MD1; Ostrosky-Zeichner, Luis MD2; Thomas, Eric J. MD, MPH1,3
Author Information

ACG Case Reports Journal 6(9):p e00208, September 2019. | DOI: 10.14309/crj.0000000000000208
     OPEN

Metrics

Abstract

Information on auto-brewery syndrome is limited in the medical literature. This rare syndrome occurs when yeast overgrowth leads to ethanol fermentation in the gut. We present a patient presenting with symptoms of alcohol intoxication with objective laboratory data of elevated blood ethanol levels without a history of alcohol consumption. We reviewed the literature and have discussed the current diagnostic and therapeutic options.

INTRODUCTION

There is limited information in the medical literature on auto-brewery syndrome, also known as gut-fermentation syndrome.1 This rare syndrome occurs because of yeast overgrowth in the gut, leading to fermentation of ethanol, thereby causing symptoms similar to alcohol intoxication without ingestion of alcohol.1 We present a patient with auto-brewery syndrome and review the available literature, including published case reports on the syndrome.

CASE REPORT

A 25-year-old white man, with no medical history or previous surgeries, presented with a chief complaint of "drunk without drinking." Two months ago, the patient noticed that he would feel very drunk after drinking his usual one or two 12-ounce beers in the evenings. This progressed to feeling drunk even when fully abstaining from alcohol. He continued to feel this way 1–2 times per week until his wife decided to bring him to the emergency department (ED) during one of his "attacks." His wife described his symptoms as slurred speech, fatigue, stumbling, dizziness, and nausea. He would eventually "pass out" and wake up in the morning with no further symptoms. His symptoms were somewhat acute and often occur in the evenings, but without any identifiable trigger. On further review, he had recently started a ketosis diet for weight loss. He did not take any over-the-counter or prescription medications. His physical examination was unremarkable with normal vital signs. Although symptomatic during a previous visit to the ED, he had a full workup including a urine drug screen, basic metabolic panel, liver function tests, complete blood count, and thyroid studies, all of which were unremarkable. He did, however, have an elevated lactic acid level of 20 mg/dL and a blood alcohol concentration of 0.3 g/dL (also elevated on a subsequent ED visit) in the absence of alcohol consumption. His symptoms improved, and he was sent home with no further treatment.

In the outpatient setting, he saw a gastroenterologist and an endocrinologist, who conducted a celiac disease workup, basic stool studies with culture, thyroid, and hypoglycemia workup, all of which were unrevealing. His wife opted to buy a breathalyzer and found that in the absence of alcohol consumption and while asymptomatic, he would score from 0.04% to 0.07%. His wife served as a control and scored 0% during these occasions. Each time the patient had symptoms, he would test at an elevated alcohol concentration, often in the 0.2% range. Based on the above workup, other etiologies were ruled out and a working diagnosis of auto-brewery syndrome was made. Subsequently, the patient was given an empiric trial of oral fluconazole 100 mg daily for 3 weeks to treat this presumed syndrome, in addition to continuing his normal diet. On completion of his therapy, the patient reported his symptoms completely resolved, with no further episodes on follow-up 4 weeks later.

DISCUSSION

Data are limited on auto-brewery syndrome, also known as gut fermentation syndrome.[1] Xiaodi et al allude to approximately

58 described cases with a large proportion being from Japan.1 There are no clear identifiable risk factors; however, Kaji et al noticed an association with previous abdominal surgeries and structural or functional disturbances, such as a dilated duodenum that can cause stagnant contents, possibly giving a favorable site for abnormal proliferation of the causative organism.2 One case reported a possible risk factor of antibiotic use, as well as a reported coinfection with Helicobacter pylori.3,4 Probiotics may also alter normal bowel flora, and although the role in this syndrome is unclear, it has been reported to predispose to Saccharomyces fungemia.5,6 There was no discussion of ethanol fermentation in these patients; however, it is possible that probiotics could predispose patients to Saccharomyces proliferation. Many case reports were able to identify a causative pathogen, often by gastric aspirations, duodenal fluid, or fecal cultures.1 Kaji et al identified that the most common organisms involved in "auto-brewery syndrome" were Candida spp. and Sacchharomyces.2

That article was to provide context on our "live-in guest" and our relationship to alcohol, not to mention our extra glycolytic tissue. There is so much more we need to learn and clearly these guys 4,000 years ago were ahead of us.

The medical papyri from Ancient Egypt is flush with "cures" that have different types of feces mixed in them. The medical papyri from Ancient Egypt is flush with "cures" that have different types of beers mixed in them. Feces carries what we today call probiotics, the beers are yeast based and they protect the microbiome.

We aren't gonna unravel this mystery in this book, we aren't even attempting to LOL... We are though making clear that the hard breathing you do after a good sprint, is a requirement not a bonus thing or a "when I get some free time thing"... Where is the alcohol and other waste products of all these bacteria that live in us going? Studies say over 5,000 different types of microbes live in our gut, totaling over 100 trillion microbes. The waste including alcohol goes where?

Where does the waste from over 100 trillion cells go?

I mean the obvious is poop, they already live in your digestive system, however... How much of their waste gets into the circulatory system? Just remember the Bible said... God made you from the dust of the ground! Iron is from that dust (space first but...), the other components from the dust are in the blood, why wouldn't microbes be?

The Healthy Human Blood Microbiome: Fact or Fiction?

Diego J Castillo 1, Riaan F Rifkin 1 2, Don A Cowan 1, Marnie Potgieter 1

Affiliations expand

PMID: 31139578 PMCID: PMC6519389 DOI: 10.3389/fcimb.2019.00148

Abstract

The blood that flows perpetually through our veins and arteries performs numerous functions essential to our survival. Besides distributing oxygen, this vast circulatory system facilitates nutrient transport, deters infection and dispenses heat throughout our bodies. Since human blood has traditionally been considered to be an entirely sterile environment, comprising only blood-cells, platelets and plasma, the detection of microbes in blood was consistently interpreted as an indication of infection. However, although a contentious concept, evidence for the existence of a healthy human blood-microbiome is steadily accumulating. While the origins, identities and functions of these unanticipated micro-organisms remain to be elucidated, information on blood-borne microbial phylogeny is gradually increasing. Given recent advances in microbial-hematology, we review current literature concerning the composition and origin of the human blood-microbiome, focusing on bacteria and their role in the configuration of both the diseased and healthy human blood-microbiomes. Specifically, we explore the ways in which dysbiosis in the supposedly innocuous blood-borne bacterial microbiome may stimulate pathogenesis. In addition to exploring the relationship between blood-borne bacteria and the development of complex disorders, we also address the matter of contamination, citing the influence of contaminants on the interpretation of blood-derived microbial datasets and urging the routine analysis of laboratory controls to ascertain the taxonomic and metabolic characteristics of environmentally-derived contaminant-taxa.

STEPPING

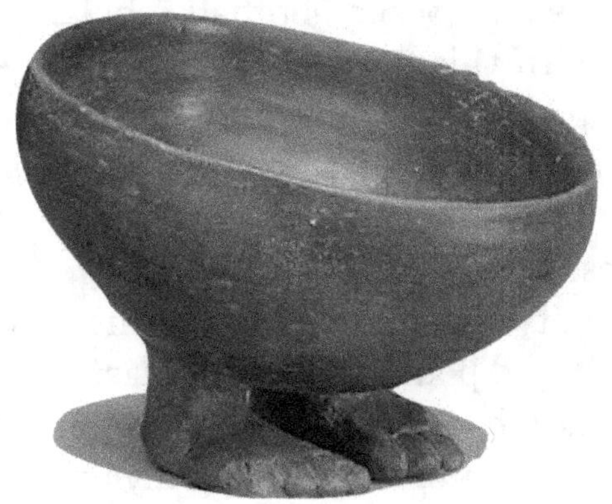

The above picture is very interesting but instead of me speaking I will provide the captioned quote from the Met Museum. You can think about this mystery as you read this chapter. We will look at this again later...

Bowl with Human Feet

What is this made of?

Pottery

When was this made?

ca. 3700–3450 B.C.

Where was this made?

Africa; Egypt

Discover

This small, round bowl sits on top of two sturdy feet. It is shaped like an Egyptian hieroglyph that looks like a small vessel with two legs and means "to bring" or "to offer." Long ago, it may have been used to bring libations, or liquid offerings, for a deity. Or it may have been used at a tomb, to make an offering of water to the deceased. The belly of the bowl tips forward, ready to pour out its contents.

Imagine

Ancient Egyptians believed that depictions could magically come alive. What would this bowl with human feet do if it came to life?

- Met Museum

Before we let some halfcocked goofball Scholars or Egyptologists have their way with this... we need to put some other eyeballs on this! Knowing that the Egyptian Gods were the powers that created or sustained life, what could this "vessel" symbolize? Maybe we should check out the feet before you make your educated guesses...

The situation that started me down this line of study was personal. I myself had plantar fasciitis (briefly) and a petite amie of mine some years back who I won't name here, had it bad... The point is I had to figure this out and my findings went waaaay beyond the feet!

Plantar Fasciitis - inflammation of a thick band of tissue that runs across the bottom of each foot and connects the heel bone to the toes, known as the plantar fascia. The cheat code is noticing that it starts with your first steps after waking up and then gets easier (damn near disappears) throughout the day. This tells you it has something to do with muscle use and/or blood flow!

This is important because this is how the Fascia work!!! This is happening everywhere throughout your body just you don't have to walk on the other tissue so you don't feel the stickiness of the tissues breaking up. The crazy part is runners and couch potatoes get it, people extremely in shape and extremely out of shape. Why? Our research says because we have not understood the fascia and it's true relationship to the body. Please read or reread L'Goat Book, particularly the section on the weighing of the Heart Ceremony.

These are feathers we are dealing with, if we think about feathers we will get this. There is more to the Horus and Hawk relationship, our body is kinda made outta feathers... crazy as it sounds! Plantar Fasciitis is our tool to learn more about the Fascia, so we need to get a working idea of the muscles in the foot and how blood flow works there. This is obviously apart of our diabetes conversation since most amputations are below the ankle. Imagine if we could stop some amputations!

The foot has 19 muscles, very similar to the spine. The adult spine has 26 vertebrae but 7 are cervical so only 19 in the body. The foot has 29 muscles but 10 come from the leg, only 19 are intrinsic to the foot.

The 10 muscles from the outside of the foot handle the big stuff like tilting the foot side to side, inversion is tilting the foot inward towards the middle of the body, eversion is tilting the foot outwards towards the hands. Stepping, the main movement we exercise with toe raises etc... Planting the foot down to lift the body up, plantar flexion. The back (dorsal) of the foot or heal flex or basically the opposite of plantar flexion is dorsiflexion. If you stand flat foot and lift the front of your foot up, that's dorsiflexion. The (19) muscles in the foot handle the movements relative to the foot. The (10) leg muscles in the foot handle the movements relative to the whole body.

There are two pillar type muscles at the back of the foot, that stabilize the leg muscles entering the foot, the extensor digitorum (digit - toe or finger) brevis and the extensor hallucis (hallux - big toe) brevis.

The hallucis extends the big toe and the digitorum extends the 4 toes (digits).

The abductor hallucis is the bulky muscle on the inside of the foot. This muscle handles the abduction and flexion of the big toe.

Abduction - moving away from the body.

Adduction - moving towards the body.

Flexion - decreases a angle. Flexion is a bending movement that decreases the angle between a segment and its proximal segment.

Extension - increases a angle. Extension is the opposite of flexion, a straightening movement that increases the angle between body parts.

The flexor digitorum brevis sits in the middle of the sole, lateral to the abductor hallucis. This muscle controls the flexion of the other 4 toes.

The abductor digiti minimi runs along the outside of the foot on the pinky toe side. This muscle is for abduction and flexion of the pinky toe.

The quadratus plantar is a oblong square-ish muscle. The muscle helps flexion of the toes.

The lumbricals (4 muscles) run along the bones of the 4 toes. Lumbricus means earth worm, kinda of clue to 'screwing in', the form and function model... These muscles work on the joints of the toes.

The flexor hallucis brevi runs along the bone of the big toe. This muscle helps flexion of the big toe.

The adductor hallucis runs across the toes. This muscle supports the arch of the foot and adduction of the big toe.

The flexor digiti minimi brevis runs along the bone of the pinky toe. The muscle helps with flexion of the pinky toe.

There are 3 plantar interossei muscles are located between the bones of the 4 toes. These muscles help adduction of the toes and joints.

There are 4 dorsal interossei muscles located between the toes. The muscles help abduction of the toes and joints.

Obviously if we are taking the time to deal with it, you know Plantar Fasciitis is associated the Diabetes. I mean the whole world can almost be classified as pre-diabetic, in really good shape (joggers or runners) or out of shape people. Then on top of those 3 types of people that almost every fits into, there is the people who sit down for 3-4 hours straight daily or more than 6 hours off and on daily. This means almost everyone!

Jumping Rope is the GOAT when it comes to this, and when it

comes to stimulating circulation. If you can't jump rope, you can fake it, just jump up and down in your house (or wherever).

When you exercise the muscles in skeletal muscle, blood flow increases to those muscles. If you have been studying your Time Tables from the AlgaRhythm and L'Goat books, you will know how much blood there is. Point is, to divert blood flow to any specific area of the body must take some away from somewhere else.

Blood flow is diverted from your core (abdominal viscera and kidneys) towards the skeletal muscle. The Heart and the worked muscle go through the motions of contracting and relaxing (we speak to the details in Melanin vs Diabetes book three the Fiscal Edition).

The particular keys that need to be noted here are EPO & N.O.. These are the two major keys to creating the 'Fountain of Youth' effect we discussed in the Was is the Aorta book. There are 3 layers of cells to the arteries and the inner layer of endothelial cells is activated by the muscle layer, which is activated by exercise!

Erythropoietin (/ɪˌrɪθroʊˈpɔɪ.ɪtɪn, -rə-, -pɔɪˈɛtɪn, -ˈiːtɪn/;[1][2][3] EPO), also known as erythropoetin, haematopoietin, or haemopoietin, is a glycoprotein cytokine secreted mainly by the kidneys in response to cellular hypoxia; it stimulates red blood cell production (erythropoiesis) in the bone marrow. - wiki

The blood leaving the kidney during exercise help create the signal that EPO is needed. EPO is known as the Master Steroid and many athletes attempt to use EPO as it is hard to detect this steroid. EPO boost every area of physical performance! The cheat code is you can make this on your own and if you've read Osiris, Diabetes and Respiration... you know whats happening with the respiratory membrane (alveolar wall, basement membrane & capillary wall).

Testosterone & Estrogen are also apart of this cycle. The Aorta & Arteries are muscles, Testosterone builds and constricts muscle, Estrogen breaks down and relaxes muscle. This could be a game changer for gyno!

Nitric oxide and its relationship to thrombotic disorders

J E Freedman 1, J Loscalzo
Affiliations expand

PMID: 12871317 DOI: 10.1046/j.1538-7836.2003.00180.x
Free article

Abstract

Nitric oxide (NO) is released by the endothelium preventing platelet adhesion to the vessel wall. When released by platelets, NO inhibits further recruitment of platelets to a growing thrombus. Modulation of endogenous NO release may be a mechanism by which the thrombotic response can be regulated as suggested by several clinical diseases associated with impaired bioactive NO. Diseases including atrial fibrillation and coronary atherothrombotic disease have been associated with impaired NO release or decrease in NO bioavailability.

Do you see what that article says??!!! Blood clots almost require the absence of Nitric Oxide to form!!!

Lets look at some Cheat Codes for the Kidneys, reason being Kidney health is key to Artery Health and Fountain of Youth function. Take note that every exercise works the Heart and the Kidney.

Avoid Tylenol/Asprin and the likes (if you can)
Avoid Bovine Serum Proteins (Dairy/Meat)
Avoid *Histamine Rich Foods which put holes in the Digestive System
Avoid Sugarery & Oily (no matter what oil) Foods
Do!! Go on a GREEN JUICE fast with Lemons!!!!
NO SPINACH
NO SEAFOOD
NO FLESH
Yes Just Juice!!! NO FOOD!!
Clogged Kidneys must be allowed to drain before whats clogging them begins to rot and putrefy,
creating infections

***L-Carnitine** - Oxidation of Sugars/Starches/Fats, its like DRAINO but it turns the waste into Electrons

Vit K - Binding proteins

Vit D - Calcium & other mineral metabolism

Vit C - soft tissue Health

Selenium/Glutathione - Antioxidant Support

Arginine (Citrulline is better) & Sunlight - N.O. production

Rehmannia (Herb and/or Tea) - Fluid Production

Molybdenum/Manganese - Creates Enzymes that dissolves Uric Acid, Sulfur, Purines & Oxalates

CoEnzyme A (liver) - Fat Burner

Ursolic Acid - Breaks Down White Adipocytes & Helps Feed Brown Adipocytes and Myocytes

Vit C - Breaks down Uric Acid, AntiOxidant

Lithium - Destroys Uric Acid & its associated symptoms (rubidium catalyzes lithium) Cherry Juice Concentrate and Celery work well however Grapefruit are Rich in Both Lithium & Vit C

Glutathione - When the body is AntiOxidant negative it will circulate Uric Acid as a AntiOxidant Substitute

Magnesium - Breaks Down and prevents Oxalates/Calcium Stones

Potassium/Citrus/Lithium - prevent crystallization of Acids/Minerals, Lemons not Grapefruits as they have oxalates

Tannins - Fights Struvite Stones

Vit D - Allows proper assimilation of Calcium, Strontium, Phosphorus & Boron)

Calcium - Yes Stones can be a sign of Deficiency, SYNTHETIC OR

NON-PLANT BASED calcium can cause stones!!!

Generally un-utilized Calcium or Calcium pulled from Bones Binds to Oxalates and causes Stones...

What do you think this bowl could mean? Keep in mind that the Gods were the powers that create or sustain life...

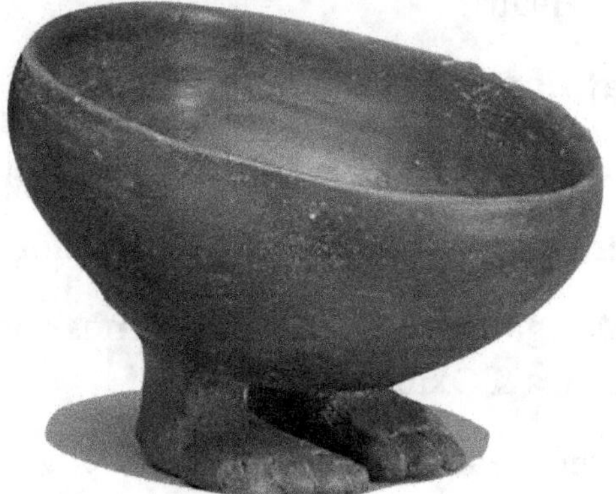

LACTIC ACID

Apart of our theory on the muscle being a digestive organ, is the fact that the skeletal muscle & heart have a low blood flow compared to metabolic rate. In comparison the kidneys and the pineal gland have relatively high blood flows compared to metabolic rate.

Mitochondria need to make an appearance in this blood story. In the Osiris, Diabetes & Respiration book we discuss Nitrogen being a crucial aspect of breathing. Our bodies were not designed, not to walk, our blood flow is completely dependent on movement. The arteries are muscles that atrophy without use...

Nitrogen in our lungs helps maintain volume pressure and without Nitric Oxide, blood CAN NOT properly carry oxygen. The pressure in the capillaries (where most amputations are formed) depends on blood flow (water structuring) and oxygen consumption, at least in relationship to oxygen diffusing into the Mitochondria.

It is a fact that the blood flow to the muscle increases exponentially for exercises. Prime example for our discussion is walking, on average blood flow to the muscles must increase 20x, just to walk wherever. Excess lactate acid production, slow removal, hypercapnia or hypoxia of any sort will hinder "the ability to perform work".

Power - rate at which work is done or energy is transformed in an electrical circuit. (Keep in mind the **Was Sceptre** is supposed to represent power and dominion of death).

If the body is electric we must step into that reality and begin to "observe" and address electrical issues. Our batteries not getting a complete charge should be clear. The liver and kidney have to run clean up on exercise, the lactic acid winds up in the blood and gets converted back into glucose! Soreness is not based on lactic acid as much as the micro tears in the muscle. Fatigue and endurance on the other hand, with the hidden master of death H2O2 (Set) is tied to lactic acid. Please read or reread the Horus & Set Transaction.

The micro tears created by exercise is healed via the relocation of the nuclei, autophagy and nutrient dense blood. The Enqi Cycle is the background energy source to facilitate the primary, especially when arteries begin to atrophy the cells have their own small reserve until power can be restored.

This is also key to sexual health and sexual performance! The power of life and death, or rebirth. Male infertility and female infertility may also be apart of this incomplete understanding we have regarding the heart and circulation.

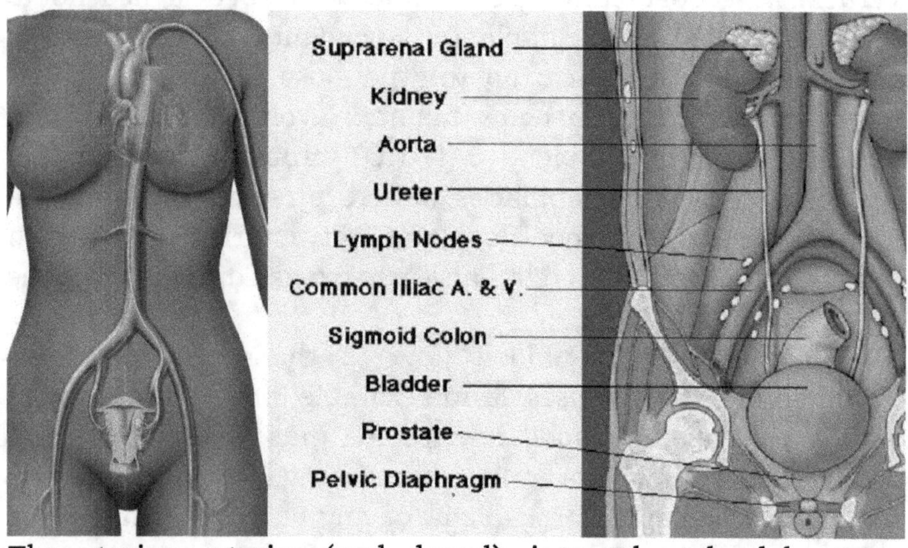

The uterine arteries (and dorsal), internal pudendal artery, inferior vesicle artery, the prostatic plexus, the ovarian artery... All these arteries are tied to this very same process! There are countless illnesses/diseases that may unknowingly be tied to H2O2, hypercapnia, hypoxia etc... These are the causes of vessel atrophy! Even the heart has a circulatory system! Remember we discussed the Vasa Vasorum (vessels of vessels)... This is all linked to circulation and the EnQi Cycle

Uterine Blood flow suffers the same way with bad food and poor exercise.... Exercise-induced blood vessel formation is known to occur in response to growth-stimulating proteins released by muscles under strain. Sirtuins, however, appears to be the key messengers relaying growth-factor signals from muscles (myokines) to blood vessels, the study found.

Modulatory Effect of Myokines on Reactive Oxygen Species in Ischemia/Reperfusion

Márton Richárd Szabó,1,2 Márton Pipicz,1,2 Tamás Csont,1,2 and Csaba Csonka1,2,3,*
Author information Article notes Copyright and License information PMC Disclaimer

Abstract

There is a growing body of evidence showing the importance of physical activity against acute ischemic events in various organs. Ischemia/reperfusion injury (I/R) is characterized by tissue damage as a result of restriction and subsequent restoration of blood supply to an organ. Oxidative stress due to increased reactive oxygen species formation and/or insufficient antioxidant defense is considered to play an important role in I/R. Physical activity not only decreases the general risk factors for ischemia but also confers direct anti-ischemic protection via myokine production. Myokines are skeletal muscle-derived cytokines, representing multifunctional communication channels between the contracting skeletal muscle and other organs through an endocrine manner. In this review, we discuss the most prominent members of the myokines (i.e., brain-derived neurotrophic factor (BDNF), cathepsin B, decorin, fibroblast growth factors-2 and -21, follistatin, follistatin-like, insulin-like growth factor-1;

interleukin-6, interleukin-7, interleukin-15, irisin, leukemia inhibitory factor, meteorin-like, myonectin, musclin, myostatin, and osteoglycin) with a particular interest in their potential influence on reactive oxygen and nitrogen species formation or antioxidant capacity. A better understanding of the mechanism of action of myokines and particularly their participation in the regulation of oxidative stress may widen their possible therapeutic use and, thereby, may support the fight against I/R.

Keywords: cardioprotection, brain, myocardial, ROS, conditioning, remote, exercise, FGF, IGF, LIF

1. Introduction

Tissue damage caused by ischemia/reperfusion (I/R) injury is presented in various clinical manifestations (e.g., myocardial infarction, stroke, peripheral arterial disease, ischemic nephropathy, etc.) and is considered to be a leading cause of death all over the world. Therefore, investigation of the potential anti-ischemic mechanisms, compounds, and strategies to attenuate I/R injury are extensively studied due to their great clinical importance [1,2].

I/R injury is characterized by tissue damage as a result of restriction and subsequent restoration of blood supply to an organ. During ischemia, oxygen and nutrient deprivation leads to time-dependent cell death [2]. The early restoration of blood flow salvages ischemic tissue and prevents complete damage; nevertheless, the reperfusion induces additional cell death to the ischemic organ damage [2]. Accumulation of reactive oxygen species (ROS) and the consequent oxidative stress prominently contribute to the cell death in I/R injury.

1.1. ROS in I/R Injury

ROS are oxygen-containing reactive molecules generated in biological systems mostly by reduction in molecular oxygen [3]. The most important representatives of ROS are superoxide anion, hydrogen peroxide (H_2O_2), and hydroxyl radical. Reactive nitrogen species (RNS) contain nitrogen, and these molecules are usually derivatives of nitric oxide (NO) or peroxynitrite (ONOO -). ROS/RNS can be either free radicals (e.g., superoxide, hydroxyl radical, NO) or non-radical reactive species (e.g., H2O2, ONOO–). ROS/RNS can be generated by either enzymatic or non-enzymatic processes. Enzymatic ROS/RNS formation include the leakage of superoxide anion from mitochondrial electron transport chain, superoxide anion production via nicotinamide adenine dinucleotide phosphate (NADPH) oxidases (NOX), xanthine oxidase, cyclooxygenases, uncoupled NO synthase (NOS), and production of NO by NOS. Non-enzymatic formation of ROS/RNS includes the generation of hydroxyl radicals from H2O2 in the Fenton or Haber–Weiss reactions or the formation of ONOO – via the rapid reaction of NO and superoxide anion. Endogenous antioxidants are important ROS scavengers that are responsible for maintaining ROS/RNS at normal levels. Both small molecules, such as glutathione and urate, or enzymatic systems, including superoxide dismutase (SOD), catalase, glutathione peroxidase (GPx), glutathione reductase, and heme oxygenase (HO), are effective components of cellular antioxidant mechanisms [3,4,5]. Oxidative stress is considered to play an important role in I/R injury, based on the findings that ROS is elevated in I/R, scavenging ROS protects against I/R injury, and experimental generation of ROS causes similar tissue damage to I/R (for review see [1,2,6,7]). Tissue nitro-oxidative stress develops in I/R injury as a result of excess formation or insufficient removal of ROS and/or RNS. Oxidative burst mainly occurs in reperfusion; nevertheless, ischemia is also accompanied by ROS production [2,8]. Besides, ischemia-induced enzymatic alterations and metabolic consequences promote oxidative burst at the beginning of reperfusion. Ischemia leads to diminished electron flux through the mitochondrial respiratory chain, which, in turn, causes superoxide anion formation at complex I and III [2], and results in the accumulation of reducing equivalents [8]. During the ischemic period, the xanthine oxidase substrate hypoxanthine is raised, and hypoxia inhibitory factor-1α is induced, which activates NOX [1,2,7]. Moreover, in response to hypoxia, xanthine dehydrogenase is converted to xanthine oxidase, and the NOS cofactor tetrahydrobiopterin is oxidized to dihydrobiopterin, resulting in the uncoupling of NOS [1,2,7]. At the beginning of reperfusion, the reintroduction of oxygen enhances the ROS generation, called the oxygen paradox [2]. Upon reperfusion, the accumulated reducing metabolites serve as electron donors for ROS formation in the mitochondrial respiratory chain [8]. In the presence of oxygen, xanthine oxidase converts hypoxanthine to xanthine, accompanied by the release of superoxide anion and hydrogen peroxide as well [1,2,7]. Uncoupled NOS and activated NOX enzymes also generate superoxide anion during reoxygenation [1,2,7]. Finally, the imbalance in the pro- and antioxidant systems leads to elevated ROS/RNS that may result in oxidative stress (i.e., oxidative damage of proteins, nucleic acids, and lipids) and can trigger activation of cell death pathways [1,2,7].

Modulation of I/R-associated oxidative stress by inhibiting ROS production and/or by enhancing antioxidant capacity seems to be a promising strategy to attenuate I/R injury and induce tissue protection [1,6,9]. For instance, inhibition of xanthine oxidase by allopurinol or the NOX enzyme by diphenyliodonium may exert protection against I/R injury in different tissues [1,7]. Furthermore, several gain or loss of function studies implicated the protective role of SOD-1 (cytosolic CuZnSOD), SOD-2 (mitochondrial MnSOD), and SOD-3 (extracellular CuZnSOD) in I/R injury [1]. Although many experimental studies focusing on oxidative stress modulation are promising, controversial preclinical findings exist, and clinical translational barriers should be overcome [1,7].

1.2. Exercise-Induced Remote Organ Protection Against I/R

Enormous effort is devoted to developing approaches limiting oxidative stress and I/R-related morbidity and mortality [9,10]. The cardiovascular beneficial effect of physical activity is well known [11,12,13]. Besides the alteration of general cardiovascular risk factors (e.g., high blood pressure or hypercholesterolemia), exercise confers direct protection against I/R injury of a distant organ. This protective effect may include the development of collateral arteries, alterations in circulation, expression of endoplasmic reticulum stress proteins, and the modulation of cyclooxygenase-2 activity, heat shock proteins, and ATP-sensitive potassium channels [14,15]. Exercise also induces antioxidant effects [16,17,18] and diminishes the increased susceptibility of cardiac mitochondria to undergo permeability transition pore opening [19]. These protective phenomena collectively are also called exercise-induced conditioning [20]. In skeletal muscle, the active use of the contractile apparatus, i.e., physical work or exercise training, leads to the release of a high amount of different skeletal muscle-derived humoral factors (e.g., myokines, metabolites, non-coding regulatory RNAs, exosomes, etc.) to regulate a variety of metabolic and cellular processes in various tissues and organs of the body, including the adipose tissue, bone, brain (central nervous system), pancreas, liver, gastrointestinal system, heart, and even the skeletal muscle itself. The collective term 'myokine 'was established by Pedersen in 2003 to be used for cytokines, which are produced and released by contracting skeletal muscles, exerting their effects in other organs of the body [21,22] through endocrine signaling pathways. The majority of myokines were also shown to exert protection against ischemia [20]. Moreover, the release of several muscle-derived myokines has been observed in settings of remote ischemic preconditioning, further emphasizing the promising beneficial role of myokines in I/R injury [23,24,25,26,27].

In this article, we aimed to review the impact of a set of relevant myokines [28,29] on the modulation of ROS formation in the context of I/R in various organs. We believe that providing a recent update and a systematic discussion of this topic may contribute to a better understanding of this field and may potentiate further research focusing on the possible use of myokines against I/R injury [23].

2. Modulatory Role of Myokines on ROS in the Context of I/R

We have performed a preliminary search using the PubMed database, and the results are presented in Table 1. First, we applied the name of certain myokines alone (column 2) as a search term or extended the search with the addition of the search term 'myokine '(column 3). Then, myokines (column 1) and 'ischemia 'were searched (column 4) to check the possible involvement of the myokines in this field. Finally, we extended this latter search with the addition of the expressions "ROS", "ROI", "oxidative", "antioxidative", "reactive", "nitric", and "stress", respectively (columns 5–11). Based on these search results, the myokines could be classified into three categories: (i) no or very weak documented associations between myokines and ischemia (for instance, in case of meteorin-like, musclin, or osteoglycin, etc.); (ii) myokines showing a marked association with ischemia and ROS (e.g., fibroblast growth factor-21 (FGF-21), irisin, leukemia inhibitory factor (LIF), etc.), and (iii) myokines with an overwhelming number of search counts, e.g., brain-derived neurotrophic factor (BDNF), fibroblast growth factor-2 (FGF-2), insulin-like growth factor-1 (IGF-1), and interleukin-6 (IL-6). However, this latter group may show deceptive values since these myokines were originally identified as signaling molecules released by non-muscular cells; for instance, IL-6 is also a well-known pro-inflammatory cytokine secreted independently from the skeletal muscle. Therefore, the interpretation of their ischemia/ROS connection needs further careful analysis. In the following paragraphs, we introduce the effects of the different myokines and the current position on their possible relation to the oxidative stress modulation in the context of I/R.

Table 1

Demonstration of the potential correlation between myokines and reactive oxygen species (ROS) after a Pubmed search.

Open in a separate window

Column 2: total number of articles obtained after searching for certain myokines, respectively. Column 3 and 4: we extended the search with the terms "myokine" and "ischemia", respectively. Column 5–11: column 2 + the terms "ischemia" and "ROS", "ROI", "oxidative", "antioxidative", "redox", "nitric", or "stress", respectively. Antiox: antioxidative; BDNF: brain-derived neurotrophic factor; CTSB: cathepsin B; FGF-2: fibroblast growth factor-2; FGF-21: fibroblast growth factor-21; FSTL-1: follistatin-like; IGF-1: insulin-like growth factor-1; IL-6: interleukin-6; IL-7: interleukin-7; IL-15: interleukin-15; LIF: leukemia inhibitory factor; METRLN: meteorin-like, ROI: reactive oxygen intermediates.

2.1. Interleukin (IL) 6

IL-6 is a multifunctional cytokine released into the blood circulation in response to physical activity, and it is considered to be the first myokine with pleiotropic effects on different tissues [30]. IL-6 binds to the IL-6 receptor (IL-6R) and gp130 receptor complex and activates diverse signaling pathways, including JAK/STAT3 pathway [30]. STAT3 transcription factor seems to be involved in cardioprotection and upregulates antioxidants (e.g., SOD-2, metallothionein) [31,32]. In connection, the antioxidant property of IL-6 has been proposed in some studies as well [33,34,35].

IL-6 has been found as a mediator of exercise-induced cardioprotection against myocardial I/R injury (Table 2) [36]. In line with these observations, few studies showed that IL-6 administration indeed induces cardioprotection [37,38]. An IL-6 pretreatment of 10 ng/mL protected cardiomyocytes against simulated I/R in a NO-dependent manner since the selective inhibition of NOS-2 (iNOS) abolished the protection [38]. IL-6 pretreatment increased NOS-2 expression and did not alter the NOS-1 (nNOS) and NOS-3 (eNOS) isoforms [38]. Mitochondrial function, which correlates to ROS formation, was also improved by IL-6 in a NO-dependent manner [38]. A loss-of-function study demonstrated that IL-6 has a pivotal role in ischemic preconditioning via JAK-STAT signaling and upregulation of NOS-2 and cyclooxygenase-2 (COX-2) [39]. Interestingly, McGinnis et al. showed that IL-6-mediated exercise-induced cardioprotection did not change myocardial NOS-2 or cyclooxygenase-2, and they suggested other possible downstream mechanisms [36].

Table 2

Effect of interleukin-6 (IL-6) on redox state in settings of ischemia/reperfusion injury (I/R).

Open in a separate window
COX-2: cyclooxygenase-2, DHE: Dihydroethidium assay, GSH: glutathione, HO: heme oxygenase, HSP70: heat shock protein 70, ip.: intraperitoneally, icv.: intracerebroventricularly, MDA: malondialdehyde, SOD-2: MnSOD, NF-kB: nuclear factor kappa-light-chain-enhancer of activated B cells, NOS-1, NOS-2, and NOS-3: neuronal/inducible/endothelial nitric oxide synthase, O2·-: superoxide anion, OGD: oxygen-glucose deprivation, sI/R: simulated ischemia/reperfusion, SOD: superoxide dismutase, ↑ and ↓ indicate increase and decrease, respectively; ↔ indicates no changes; * indicates the detection method.

It has been demonstrated that IL-6 is neuroprotective in cerebral ischemia [40,41,42,43], so it is plausible that exercise-induced IL-6 release contributes to the protection against ischemic stroke. In vivo administration of 50 ng IL-6 reduced cerebral infarction, restored SOD-2 expression via IL-6R-STAT3 pathway, and blocked the oxidation and dissociation of IL-6R and gp130 [40]. They suggested that the oxidation and subsequent disruption of the IL-6 receptor contribute to I/R injury and IL-6 protects against oxidative stress by preserving IL-6 receptor complex integrity and by the upregulation of antioxidants (e.g., SOD-2) [40]. Similar findings were obtained in oxygen–glucose deprivation (OGD)-primary neuronal cells treated with IL-6 [40]. In neuronal stem cells, IL-6 increased the activation of STAT3, expression of SOD-2, and decreased superoxide anion production [44]. These mechanisms were in casual relation to the cytoprotection against OGD and in vivo ischemic stroke [44].

IL-6 also seemed to participate in the protection against I/R injury in the liver and be associated with ROS modulation [45,46,47]. IL-6 treatment decreased oxidative stress–responsive HO-1 and NF-kappaB, accumulation of MDA, and increased GSH content in fatty liver subjected to I/R [47]. MnSOD (SOD-2) was increased in response to IL-6 in hypoxia/reoxygenation-exposed hepatocytes via STAT3 pathways [46]. Interestingly, Tiberio et al. suggested that Hsp70 expression may play an important role in the IL-6-induced hepatoprotection [45], partly because Hsp70 increases antioxidant GSH content by the modulation of glutathione-related enzymes [48].

2.2. Irisin

Irisin, the derivative of the fibronectin type III domain-containing protein 5 (FNDC5), was first described in 2013 [49]. Irisin is capable of inducing changes in adipose tissue [50,51] by increasing the expression of uncoupling protein-1 (UCP-1), thereby leading to the conversion of white adipose tissue to brown adipose tissue (by a process termed browning) and resulting in the formation of the beige adipose tissue. Irisin also increases thermogenesis, metabolism of lipids and glucose, and reduces adipogenesis [52,53]. The intracellular signaling pathway of browning is based on the phosphorylation of mitogen-activated protein kinases (MAPKs), such as extracellular signal-regulated kinases (ERKs) and p38 protein [50,54].

The potential protective effect of irisin in ischemia (and reperfusion), particularly in the myocardium via ROS formation, has been presented by a few papers (Table 3). Wang and colleagues found that exogenous irisin administration (100 µg/kg intraperitoneally) plays a pivotal role in protecting the heart against I/R injury by increasing SOD-1 levels in C57/BL6 mice [55]. Similarly, another study showed that 1 µg/kg intravenous administration of exogenous irisin produced dose-dependent protection against I/R-induced injury to the heart, reduced total ROS production, and simultaneously increased SOD activity [56]. They also found that in the presence of heat-denatured irisin, the protective effects on cardiac I/R injury were lost. In another paper, irisin treatment reduced the levels of ROS and increased the levels of components of the antioxidative system, including glutathione, SOD, and GPx via the dynamin-like GTPase optic atrophy 1 protein [57]. Administration of exogenous irisin also conferred protection against I/R-induced injury and oxidative stress in the lung [58]. Irisine at 12.5–50 nmol/L concentration mitigated oxygen–glucose deprivation (OGD)-induced neuronal injury and reversed OGD-induced oxidative stress in neuronal cells [59], and in a similar model, it suppressed the levels of nitrotyrosine, superoxide anion, and 4-hydroxynonenal (4-HNE) in peri-infarct brain tissues [60]. Intravenous irisin administration reduced malondialdehyde and myeloperoxidase levels but increased SOD and GPx activities in a mouse model of intestinal I/R injury [61] and significantly decreased the ROS accumulation. It decreased the levels of MDA, XO, and 4-HNT, while it increased the levels of SOD and GPx in intestinal tissues after gut I/R which was neutralized by irisin antibody [62]. Exogenous irisin significantly decreased oxidative stress in hepatic I/R [63,64,65]. Irisin given intraperitoneally at 250 µg/kg concentration reduced ER stress and oxidative stress after renal I/R, which was associated with the upregulation of GPx-4. TRSL3 (a GPx4 inhibitor) reduced the expression of GPx4 and abolished the protective effects of irisin in I/R-induced acute kidney injury, suggesting that GPx4 is a vital component in irisin's protective effect after renal I/R. [66]. Irisin administration at a concentration of 100 µg/kg increased SOD and reduced MDA levels relative to those mice in the renal I/R group, indicating that irisin has a protective effect on the kidney by inhibiting oxidative stress in I/R injury [67].

Table 3

Effect of Irisin on redox state in settings of I/R.

Open in a separate window

4-HNE: 4-hydroxynonenal, A/R: anoxia/reoxygenation, DHE: Dihydroethidium assay, GPx: glutathione peroxidase, H/R: hypoxia/reoxygenation, ip.: intraperitoneally, iv.: intravenously, MDA: malondialdehyde, SOD-1: CuZnSOD, SOD-2: MnSOD, MPO: myeloperoxidase, N.A.: not available, $O_2 \cdot^-$: superoxide anion, OGD: oxygen–glucose deprivation, ROS: reactive oxygen species, SOD: superoxide dismutase, UCP-2: mitochondrial uncoupling protein 2, XOR: xanthine oxidoreductase, ↑ and ↓ indicate increase and decrease, respectively; ↔ indicates no changes; * indicates detection method.

2.3. Brain-Derived Neurotrophic Factor (BDNF)

It is well accepted that muscle contraction-induced myokine release, particularly BDNF, has neurotrophic and neuroprotective effects [68]. The neurotrophic factor BDNF is an important regulator for the development of brain circuits, neuronal development, synaptic and neuronal network plasticity, as well as for neuroregeneration and neuroprotection and modulation of synaptic activity [69]. Independently of the neuronal properties, neurotrophins exert unique cardiovascular activities. The heart is innervated by sensory, sympathetic, and parasympathetic neurons, which require neurotrophins during early development and in the establishment of mature properties, contributing to the maintenance of cardiovascular homeostasis. The identification of molecular mechanisms that are regulated by neurotrophins and involved in the crosstalk between cardiac sympathetic nerves, cardiomyocytes, cardiac fibroblasts, and vascular cells has a fundamental importance in normal heart function and direct the response of the cardiovascular system to acute and chronic injury [70,71]. It is well accepted that BDNF acts on its downstream target receptor, the tropomyosin receptor kinase B, thereby activating the (BDNF)/TrkB pathway.

Based on a Pubmed search, a high number of hits were found for the term 'BDNF 'and 'ischemia '(1092). Therefore, we expected a lot of new or possible links between BDNF and ROS. However, only a few articles were found showing direct evidence between BDNF and ROS-induced regulation of ischemia (Table 4). González-Rodríguez and Ugidos investigated exogenous BDNF administration in ex vivo rat brain slices subjected to oxygen and glucose deprivation (OGD) models. They showed that BDNF in a concentration of 50 ng/mL given into the medium was capable of conferring neuroprotective effect and preventing oxidative stress characterized by decreased ROS production (tissue ROS production, NADPH oxidase activity, and lipid peroxidation) [72]. The direct effect of BDNF on ROS was also shown in PC12h cells. BDNF did not seem to change the total amount of ROS in the cells treated with xanthine and xanthine oxidase but increased superoxide anion and decreased H2O2 levels in neurons of the central nervous system, suggesting that reducing the conversion from superoxide anion to H2O2 is also critical for the protection by BDNF [73]. In contrast to these findings, others found that the expression and activation of NADPH oxidase were increased after a 2-day exposure to BDNF. In primary cortical cell cultures, BDNF produced oxidative stress in cortical neurons through NADPH oxidase-mediated production of superoxide anion, and BDNF induced expression and activation of NADPH oxidase, which caused oxidative neuronal necrosis [74]. A similar finding was published in human vascular endothelium: BDNF induced NOX-derived ROS generation through activation of p47 phox in a TrkB receptor-dependent manner, which led to the promotion of angiogenic tube formation possibly via Akt activation [75].

Table 4

Effect of different myokines on redox state in settings of I/R.

Open in a separate window

1 H2O2 treatment to mimic I/R, 2 7,8-DHF a BDNF mimetic, BDNF: brain-derived neurotrophic factor, 3NT: 3-nitrotyrosine, 4-HNE: 4-hydroxynonenal, 7,8-DHF: 7,8-dihydroxyflavone, 8-OHdG: 8-hydroxy-2-deoxyguanosine, NOS-3: endothelial nitric oxide synthase, FGF-2: Fibroblast growth factor 2, FGF-21: Fibroblast growth factor-21, FSTL-1: Follistatin-like 1, GPx: glutathione peroxidase, H/R: hypoxia/reoxygenation, IGF-1: Insulin-like growth factor 1, ip.: intraperitoneally, iv.: intravenously, LIF: leukemia inhibitory factor, MCAO: middle cerebral artery occlusion, MDA: malondialdehyde, N.A.: not applicable, NOX: NADPH oxidase, O2·−: superoxide anion, OGD: oxygen-glucose deprivation, Prdx4: Peroxiredoxin-4, SOD: superoxide dismutase, SOD-3: Extracellular superoxide dismutase [CuZn], TBARS: thiobarbituric acid reactive substances, ↑ and ↓ indicate increase and decrease, respectively; ↔ indicates no changes; * indicates detection method.

The potential protective role of BDNF against ischemia was proved by the BDNF mimetic 7,8-dihydroxyflavone (7,8-DHF).

Intraperitoneal administration of 5 mg/kg 7,8-DHF two days after ischemia for four weeks attenuated cardiac dysfunction and cardiomyocyte abnormality of myocardial ischemic mice. Moreover, 7,8-DHF reduced cell death, accompanied by inhibiting mitochondrial superoxide anion generation [76]. Furthermore, exercise-induced BDNF confers certain aspects of its cardioprotective effects through the activation of the BDNF/TrkB axis in a NO-dependent manner [77].

We found a lot more studies from recent years investigating the relation between BDNF and ROS in ischemia. However, these studies are less relevant, because no causative relation was demonstrated between BDNF and ROS. In all of these papers, the central nervous system or the neurons represented the endpoints of the studies, and exclusively rodent animal models (rats and mice) were used with a wide range of secondary end-points, i.e., oxidative stress [78,79,80], SOD [81,82,83], NOS [84,85], HO-1 [86,87], or others [88,89,90].

2.4. Follistatin-Like 1

Follistatin-like 1 (FSTL-1) is a TGF-β1 induced, secreted glycoprotein that belongs to the follistatin family of proteins [100]. FSTL-1 is expressed and secreted by human skeletal muscle cells after physical activity. Serum FSTL-1 level is increased after 60 min of cycling [101] and high-intensity all-out sprint interval training [102], while 11 weeks of strength training enhanced FSTL-1 mRNA expression in vastus lateralis and trapezius muscles [103]. Several articles reported the possible involvement of FSTL-1 against ischemic diseases [104,105,106]. Resistance exercise-stimulated skeletal muscle-derived FSTL-1 not only reached the heart via the circulation but also reverted post-AMI cardiac remodeling and improved cardiac angiogenesis [107,108]. Both intravenous administration and transgenic overexpression of FSTL-1 protein protected cardiomyocytes against I/R injury through the Akt/AMPK pathway with subsequent NOS-3 activation and suppressed apoptosis and inflammatory response [109,110]. However, some studies refer to FSTL-1 as a cardiokine rather than myokine, appointing the heart as the major source of circulating FSTL-1 protein since its secretion is increasing rapidly after myocardial injury [111,112]. Correspondingly, FSTL-1 derived from mesenchymal stem cells protected against I/R in vivo and in vitro, enhanced SOD activity, and decreased malondialdehyde concentration (Table 4) [92]. Furthermore, cardiac overexpression of FSTL-1 reduced the severity of doxorubicin-induced cardiocytotoxicity via restoring the decreased protein level of nuclear factor erythroid 2–related factor-2 (NRF-2), upregulating SOD-1 and SOD-2 mRNA expression and reducing myocardial ROS, malondialdehyde, and 4-hydroxynonenal levels [113]. Additionally, it was reported that circulating FSTL-1 in healthy individuals is positively correlated with derivatives of reactive oxidative metabolites [114], suggesting that FSTL-1 could be induced by oxidative stress. Regarding skeletal muscle, FSTL-1 promotes endothelial cell function and improves revascularization in ischemic hindlimbs through activation of Akt-NOS-3 signaling (Table 4) [91]. Moreover, treatment of C2C12 murine skeletal muscle cell line with inflammatory cytokines, such as interferon-γ and IL-1β enhanced FSTL-1 secretion [101].

2.5. Fibroblast Growth Factor-21

Fibroblast growth factor-21 (FGF-21) is a regulator of glucose and lipid metabolism [115] and expressed mainly in the liver [116]. Apart from its pivotal role in energy balance, FGF-21 is also synthesized [117] and even secreted by skeletal muscle after a single boost [118] and two weeks of treadmill exercise [119]. A series of studies suggested that FGF-21 exhibits diverse beneficial functions against myocardial infarction and adverse cardiac remodeling, while elevated circulating FGF-21 is also suggested to be a sensitive biomarker for the detection of I/R injury during liver transplantation [120], implying that elevation of blood FGF-21 might be considered as an endogenous adaptive response against cellular damage. Treatment of cultured cardiomyocytes and adult mice with the pro-inflammatory agent lipopolysaccharide enhanced cardiac FGF-21 protein levels resulting in upregulated expression of antioxidant genes including SOD-2 and UCP-3, as well as decreased the extent of ROS formation possibly via an autocrine manner [121]. On the other hand, FGF-21 also confers cardioprotection via an endocrine manner. Skeletal muscle-derived FGF-21 improved cardiac function reduced apoptosis and proinflammatory cytokines after myocardial infarction [122]. Furthermore, serum FGF-21 concentration is elevated after myocardial infarction. However, the major source of circulating FGF-21 is considered to be the liver and the adipose tissue [123,124]. The action of Sirtuin 1 deacetylase, which is responsible for antioxidant gene expression in cardiac tissue [125,126,127], is partially mediated by FGF-21 [121]. In line with that, in response to doxorubicin-induced oxidative stress, FGF-21 pretreatment increased the amount of cardiac Sirtuin-1, thereby preventing subsequent cellular injury [128]. The same study also revealed that pretreatment with FGF-21 suppressed chronic doxorubicin-induced 3-nitrotyrosine, 4-hydroxy-2-nonenal, and MDA levels in murine hearts. Intraperitoneal administration of recombinant human FGF-21 for 28 days enhanced both mRNA and protein levels of SOD-2 and catalase, moreover mitigated angiotensin II-induced ROS release in the murine heart [129]. Several studies implied that NRF-2 activation is essential for FGF-21 mediated antioxidant response. NRF-2 induced hepatic FGF-21 expression and secretion in obese mice [130] and even protected the liver against oxidative stress [131], while FGF-21 deficiency enhanced type 1 diabetes-induced oxidative stress in the heart [132]. Furthermore, FGF-21 supplementation prevented lipid- or diabetes-induced cardiac apoptosis and lipotoxicity-induced cardiomyopathy, possibly through inhibition of Fyn-mediated export of NRF-2 from the nucleus [133,134]. In line with that, fenofibrate treatment significantly ameliorated diabetes-induced renal oxidative stress and dysfunction, and this beneficial effect is associated with increased FGF-21 expression and subsequent activation of NRF-2 [135]. Additionally, FGF-21 treatment restored doxorubicin-induced downregulation of NRF-2, as well as its target proteins, such as NADPH quinone oxidoreductase-1, catalase, and HO-1 levels [128]. Moreover, in vitro treatment of H9C2 cardiac cell line with FGF-21 protected against H2O2-induced cell death and decreased superoxide anion formation after simulated I/R (Table 4) [93]. The proposed mechanisms for the observed cytoprotective effect might be the enhancement of autophagy and inhibition of angiopoietin-2 [136,137,138]. Another possible way of the suppression of oxidative stress induced damage is the modulation of endoplasmic reticulum (ER) stress. FGF-21 expression and secretion are increased in response to ER-stress while FGF-21 overexpression protected cardiomyocytes against ER stress [139]. Additionally, FGF-21 transcription is highly regulated by activating transcription factor 4 (ATF-4) and CCAAT enhancer-binding protein homologous protein (CHOP), two important regulators of redox homeostasis and ER-stress [140].

2.6. Decorin

The small leucine-rich proteoglycan decorin is part of the extracellular matrix and a positive regulator of muscle hypertrophy [141]. Secreted from myotubes during differentiation [142], long term, combined endurance and resistance exercise upregulated decorin mRNA in vastus lateralis muscles, also markedly elevated plasma decorin level immediately after a single boost of resistance training [141]. Beyond that, decorin may ameliorate I/R injury via reducing oxidative/nitrative stress [143]. Intraperitoneal administration of decorin before 60 min ischemia attenuated lipid peroxidation and enhanced SOD levels in the kidney (Table 4) [94]. Moreover, decorin treatment protected cultured rat cardiomyocytes exposed to simulated I/R-induced cell death [144]. In line with that, decorin conferred antioxidant properties against traumatic brain injury [145], as well as attenuated diabetes-induced cardiomyopathy and promoted angiogenesis, possibly through activating the IGF-1 receptor [146].

2.7. Myonectin

The recently identified myokine C1q and tumor necrosis factor-related protein 5, also known as myonectin, is predominantly expressed by skeletal muscle and may function as an endocrine factor [147]. Serum myonectin was increased after 8 weeks of aerobic exercise [148], while treadmill running for 4 weeks enhanced myonectin mRNA and protein content in the soleus muscle and elevated plasma myonectin level as well [149]. However, little is known about the potential modulatory effect of myonectin on I/R related oxidative damage. B6 vitamin supplementation upregulated myonectin and leukemia inhibitory factor, as well as NRF-2 mRNA expression in the gastrocnemius muscle, suggesting a potential role of myonectin in the antioxidant system [150]. Moreover, systemic administration, transgenic overexpression, and treatment of cultured myocytes with myonectin protected against ischemic injury via decreasing the rate of apoptosis and inflammation [149].

2.8. Insulin-Like Growth Factor-1 (IGF-1)

Insulin-like growth factor 1 (IGF-1) is synthesized mainly in the liver and acts as a growth and differentiation factor. IGF-1 is also synthesized by skeletal muscle after physical activity [151,152,153,154]. Apart from its prominent role in muscle hypertrophy and regeneration, IGF-1 exerts protection against oxidative stress-induced cellular injury. The dominant isoform of muscle IGF-1 minimized oxidative damage in senescent muscle via upregulating peroxisome proliferator-activated receptor gamma coactivator 1-alpha (PGC-1α), NRF-2, and Sirtuin-1 [155]. IGF-1 pretreatment of cultured rat cardiomyocytes mitigated hypoxia/reoxygenation-induced cell death, reduced subsequent oxidative stress, and inhibited MDA production (Table 4) [95]. IGF-1 overexpression suppressed the formation of H_2O_2, hydroxyl radical, and nitrotyrosine accumulation, thus protected against diabetic cardiomyopathy [156]. Likewise, attenuation of circulating IGF-1 levels, through knockout of liver-specific IGF-1, resulted in downregulated expression of NRF-2 and its downstream targets NADPH quinone oxidoreductase-1, γ-glutamylcysteine ligase, and HO-1 in the aorta [157]. Additionally, the same research group assessed that exposing cultured aorta segments from IGF-1 deficient mice to H_2O_2 or oxidized low-density lipoprotein exacerbated oxidative stress-mediated cellular injury. Controversially, isolated cardiomyocytes from hepatic IGF-1 deficient mice showed decreased ROS formation after treatment with the pro-oxidant paraquat [158]. Apart from its antioxidant properties, IGF-1 protects against I/R injury both in vivo and in vitro. Intravenous injection of IGF-1 30 min before left anterior descending artery ligation ameliorated myocardial infarct size and apoptosis [159]. Downregulation of IGF-1 during I/R through microRNA-320 and microRNA-489 aggravated the extent of myocardial infarction, ventricular remodeling, and apoptotic cell death [160,161], proposing an important IGF-1 mediated endogenous protection against ischemic cell death. This is further affirmed by the findings that genetic depletion of mouse mast cell protease 4—presumably responsible for endogenous IGF-1 degradation—alleviated myocardial infarct size, post-ischemic cardiac dysfunction and remodeling [162]. IGF-1 also confers cardioprotection in ex vivo perfused myocardium [163] since both supplementation of IGF-1 into the perfusion fluid or IGF-1 overexpression suppressed I/R injury [164,165]. Recently it was demonstrated that subcutaneous IGF-1 supplementation for 3 days improved cardiac function after myocardial infarction [166]. Transgenic overexpression of locally acting IGF-1 isoform (mIGF-1) mitigated paraquat-induced oxidative stress, alleviated cardiac MDA production, ROS levels, as well as 4-hydroxy-2-nonenal and MDA protein adducts [127,167]. The proposed mechanism may involve the activation of Sirtuin-1 deacetylase since overexpression of mIGF-1 isoform increased cardiac Sirtuin-1 protein level in both HL-1 cells and murine primary cardiomyocytes, while genetic depletion of Sirtuin-1 abolished the protection induced by mIGF-1 against paraquat-induced oxidative damage.

2.9. Leukemia Inhibitory Factor (LIF)

LIF belongs to the IL-6 cytokine superfamily, presumed as a pleiotropic cytokine with a wide range of activities, including modulation of cell proliferation and growth, bone formation, and neuronal protection. LIF mRNA expression is acutely induced after 6 h of concentric exercise in the vastus lateralis [168], thereby pointing to the skeletal muscle as a putative source of circulating LIF. Intravenous administration of LIF protected rabbit hearts against ex vivo I/R injury, moreover increased myocardial SOD-2 activity, decreased lipid oxidation, and protein carbonylation (Table 4) [96]. Additionally, LIF transfection improved cardiac recovery and enhanced the proliferation of cardiomyocytes following myocardial infarction [169]. LIF treatment mitigated middle cerebral artery occlusion [170] and focal cerebral ischemia-induced injury, in the latter via upregulating the antioxidant enzyme peroxiredoxin 4 mRNA in cultured oligodendrocytes and SOD-3 mRNA expression in cortical neurons (Table 4) [97,98]. LIF also protected PC-12 cells against Antimycin A-induced oxidative damage, reduced ROS level, and restored SOD activity [171]. Furthermore, LIF attenuated glucose-induced ROS production in podocytes, decreased NADPH oxidase generation while enhancing total SOD levels [172].

2.10. Fibroblast Growth Factor 2 (FGF-2)

FGF-2, also known as basic fibroblast growth factor, is a pleiotropic protein with important roles in angiogenesis, bone formation, cell differentiation, and migration. Despite lacking the secretion signal, the low molecular weight isoform of FGF-2 is a secreted protein [173,174]. Cultured myocytes exposed to in vitro mechanical stress or scratching responded with increased FGF-2 secretion in the surrounding media [175,176,177], proposing that FGF-2 might be an exercise-induced myokine [178]. Presumed to act via autocrine/paracrine manner, FGF-2 is well documented to protect against I/R. However, it remains controversial whether the skeletal muscle-derived secreted FGF-2 isoform is involved in cardioprotection. Cardiac-specific overexpression of FGF-2 conferred cardioprotection in the ex vivo perfused murine heart [179,180,181,182], while FGF-2 knockout failed to attenuate the extent of I/R injury [183]. Interestingly, it is proposed that the low molecular weight isoform of FGF-2 might have a prominent role in these beneficial effects on the myocardium

[184,185]. Additionally, treatment with both low and high molecular weight isoforms of FGF-2 protected cultured rat cardiomyocytes against doxorubicin-mediated oxidative stress [186], possibly via preventing the doxorubicin-induced decrease in NRF-2 and enhancing the subsequent upregulation of HO-1 [187,188]. Intraperitoneal administration of FGF-2 markedly alleviated I/R-induced kidney damage (Table 4) [99,189]. The proposed mechanism of action might involve the attenuation of mitochondrial DNA damage as reflected by lowering the amounts of 3-nitrotyrosine and 8-hydroxy-2-deoxyguanosine generation of tubular cells in ischemic kidneys and inhibition of excessive ER-stress. FGF-2 is also involved in the protection against cerebral ischemia [190] and mitigated H2O2-induced oxidative damage of PC-12 cells, possibly through mediating ER-stress response [191].

2.11. Other Myokines

In the case of 8 other myokines, i.e., cathepsin B, follistatin, IL-7, IL-15, meteorin-like, musclin, myostatin, and osteoglycin, no relevant literature was found in the context of ROS and I/R (Table 1, Figure 1). However, their potential redox modulatory role is discussed in the next section.

Modulation of ischemia/reperfusion-induced reactive oxygen species (ROS) formation and/or elimination by myokines in different organs. This figure shows the groups of myokines affecting ROS or antioxidant mechanisms in the heart, brain, liver, and kidneys, respectively, in the settings of ischemia/reperfusion (thick lines). The effect of the individual myokines on specific molecular targets are indicated with thin lines: T: negative effect, ↑ : positive effect. BDNF: brain-derived neurotrophic factor; FGF-2: fibroblast growth factor 2; FGF-21: fibroblast growth factor 21; FSTL-1: follistatin-like; GPx: glutathione peroxidase; GSH: glutathione; HO-1: heme oxygenase-1; IGF-1: insulin-like growth factor-1; IL-6: interleukin-6; IL-7: interleukin-7; IL-15: interleukin-15; LIF: leukemia inhibitory factor; METRLN: meteorin-like; NOS: nitric oxide synthase; NOX: NADPH oxidase;

ONOO–: peroxynitrite, O2.–: superoxide anion, SOD: superoxide dismutase, ROS: reactive oxygen species. ?: no article was found to support evidence between myokines and ROS. Figure 1 was created by the software Inkscape.

Go to:

3. Discussion

In summary, we found that several myokines confer protection against I/R injury in a variety of organs. This protection often involves the modulation of ROS/RNS formation or elimination (Figure 1).

We may conclude that some myokines exert significant effects on the redox homeostasis of tissues. Therefore, these mediators may potentially confer general protection against I/R injury. Irisin, IL-6, and BDNF are the most powerful members of these myokines. One may speculate that the use of these myokines in combination or application of physical exercise forms resulting in high irisin, IL-6, and BDNF-release would provide an even more pronounced preventive or therapeutic effect against ischemic stress. However, confirmation of these concepts needs to be done in future studies.

Importantly, all of the myokines that were investigated concerning ROS modulation were found to (i) decrease ROS formation and its harmful consequences (e.g., lipid peroxidation, etc.), or (ii) increase antioxidant enzymes protein level or activity. Superoxide anion was represented as the most frequent target of redox status according to the studies we analyzed, and among the antioxidative defense enzymes, SOD and GPx, were investigated most frequently. Taken together, the prooxidant effect of myokines could hardly be found concerning I/R (Table 2, Table 3 and Table 4).

Although in our preliminary PubMed search, we found a relatively large number of myokines in the context of I/R and ROS, it seems that only a portion of these myokines (9 out of 18) influences the redox balance significantly and are in a causative relationship with ROS/RNS formation or elimination. In several articles, the influence of myokines on ROS/RNS formation was only a secondary or tertiary finding. Moreover, in the case of several other myokines (i.e., cathepsin, follistatin, IL-7, IL-15, METRLN, musclin, myonectin, myostatin, osteoglycin), no or only very weak evidence was found to link the individual myokines to possible modulation of redox balance (Figure 1). This does not exclude the possibility that these myokines may be involved in the protection against I/R injury. However, further studies are required to clarify their precise role and mechanism of action.

In recent years, exercise training and other forms of physical activity have become one of the main clinical interventions for the prevention and treatment of (cardio)vascular diseases (sport as medicine). Therefore, a better understanding of the mechanisms underlying myokine release holds promise for the discovery of novel therapeutic targets and optimization of physical activity to improve (cardio)vascular outcomes.

Go to:

Abbreviations

*I know that article may have been a lot but listen BLESS SEBI'S SOUL however he may have hurt many with agave! Many that have not done their own research or followed our movement may have hurt people with agave. Fructose inhibits NAD, we have been inundated by high fructose corn syrup from the big companies and agave from sebi-ites… NAD is the key to the EnQi Cycle and Water/Melanin function in the cells!

What we are getting at here now is that the muscle is apart of breathing. The full body participates in breathing. The diaphragm is the "EnQi Cycle of breathing", what I mean is the diaphragm is the initial muscle for the lungs, however it becomes the minimum as the body continues to develop. Our theory is that the body doesn't completely develop on it's own. All of the skeletal muscle contribute to the ebb and flow of blood that controls breathing. If we take for instance the environmental phthalates that have been documented to contribute to uterine fibroids… Exercise maybe a bigger key than even what has been promoted, the problem maybe incorrect exercise... Women has more fat naturally, more chemical exposure from "beauty products" plus less exercise which is culturally accepted equals.... No Bueno!

Nitrosamines from Meat and commercial beer have to enter this conversation somewhere. Nitrosamines are proven to cause cancers! If this is in beer how do we get here from the medicinal origins of beer?

Nitrites and Nitrates behave very differently in the body, contributing factors are exercise patterns and eating habits! To put this simple in a disease forming environment nitrites become the leaders of the pack and in a life forming in-iron-ment they become supporters of life. Nitrites are very unstable, they don't have a mind of their own. Oxygen is the stabilizing force here, NO2 being nitrite has one less oxygen than the NO3 of nitrate.

Here is where the rubber meets the road, low PH combined with bad bacteria (or good bacteria gone rogue) or inflammation... The key is the nutrients we discuss in the June July book protect the digestive system from this process. Please read and/or reread that book!

BITTERS

Before we just go right to the journals, here we are pointing out that the Heart & the Aorta have receptors for Bitter Herbs.... If you know me though you know I have that GOAT look on my face bwahahahahahaha...

Of course they knew this in Ancient Egypt, the medical papyri attest to this!!! Beer and Bread are almost identical recipes too... Just a FYI...

Extraoral bitter taste receptors in health and disease

Ping Lu,1 Cheng-Hai Zhang,1 Lawrence M. Lifshitz,2,3 and Ronghua ZhuGe1,2
Author information Article notes Copyright and License information PMC Disclaimer

Go to:
ABSTRACT
Bitter taste receptors (TAS2Rs or T2Rs) belong to the superfamily of seven-transmembrane G protein–coupled receptors, which are the targets of >50% of drugs currently on the market. Canonically, T2Rs are located in taste buds of the tongue, where they initiate bitter taste perception. However, accumulating evidence indicates that T2Rs are widely expressed throughout the body and mediate diverse nontasting roles through various specialized mechanisms. It has also become apparent that T2Rs and their polymorphisms are associated with human disorders. In this review, we summarize the physiological and pathophysiological roles that extraoral T2Rs play in processes as diverse as innate immunity and reproduction, and the major challenges in this

emerging field.

Introduction

"Good medicine always tastes bitter." This ancient Oriental wisdom may soon be verified with modern biology. Traditionally, bitter taste, one of five basic taste qualities, is thought to guide organisms to avoid harmful toxins and noxious substances and thus is critical to animal and human survival. The sensors for bitter compounds in vertebrates are bitter taste receptors (T2Rs or TAS2Rs), a class of G protein–coupled receptors (GPCRs) originally identified in type II taste receptor cells in the taste bud. Traditionally it has been assumed that, responding to the pressure of food selection, different species have evolved with different numbers of T2Rs: 25 in humans and 35 in mice (Shi et al., 2003; Chandrashekar et al., 2006). Over the past decade, however, the expression of T2Rs and their downstream signaling molecules have been found in several extraoral systems, including the digestive, respiratory, and genitourinary systems, as well as in brain and immune cells. Moreover, these receptors carry out different biological functions in their varied locations. These findings raise the intriguing possibilities that the evolution of T2Rs may also be influenced by the biological functions mediated by these receptors in the extraoral cells and tissues (Campbell et al., 2014), that these extraoral T2Rs may be attractive targets for new medicines, and that currently used bitter medicines may exert their pharmacological functions by acting on these extraoral receptors—which, until now, have been considered side effects or adverse effects.

In this review, we summarize our current understanding of bitter tasting in extraoral systems and the roles that extraoral T2Rs play in processes as diverse as innate immunity, secretion, contraction, reproduction, and urination. We also summarize the association of T2R polymorphisms with various disorders and the roles of T2Rs in abnormal conditions. As this is an emerging area and our understanding is still rudimentary, we discuss the obstacles that the field is encountering and offer our perspective on how to overcome them.

T2R signaling cascades

The canonical T2R signal transduction cascade shares common signaling molecules with sweet and umami receptors (i.e., T1Rs; Kautiainen, 1992; Wong et al., 1996; Huang et al., 1999; Chandrashekar et al., 2000; Mueller et al., 2005), which include heterotrimeric G protein subunits (i.e., α-gustducin [Gnat3], Gβ3, and Gγ13), a phospholipase C (PLCβ2), an inositol trisphosphate receptor (InsP3R), and a transient receptor potential cation channel (TRPM5; Fig. 1, A and B). Upon receptor activation, the G protein gustducin dissociates its α, Gnat3, and βγ subunits. The latter activates PLCβ2, leading to a release of Ca2+ from InsP3-sensitive Ca2+ stores and resulting in Na+ influx through TRPM5 channels. This Na+ influx depolarizes the cells and causes the release of neurotransmitter ATP through gap junction hemichannels or CALHM1 ion channels (Finger et al., 2005; Chaudhari and Roper, 2010; Taruno et al., 2013). Finally, released ATP activates purinergic receptors on nerves in the taste buds, and the resulting impulse is transmitted to the taste center in the central nervous system to initiate the perception of bitter taste (Taruno et al., 2013; Peng et al., 2015).

The canonical T2R signaling pathway. (A) The invariant portion of T2R-mediated signaling in the tongue and extraoral cells/ tissues includes bitter compounds binding (outside the cell; not depicted) with the receptors to increase intracellular calcium. (B) The remaining components of the T2R pathway in the taste bud.

In contrast, nonlingual T2Rs use at least three different mechanisms to execute biological roles tailored to their location. These three cascades have the same initial half (i.e., beginning from receptor activation to the increase in intracellular calcium concentration [[Ca2+]i]) as the canonical T2R signaling cascade (Fig. 1 A) and subsequently diverge to result in diverse functions in different cell types or tissues. These three mechanisms can be called cell-autonomous regulation, paracrine regulation, and endocrine regulation.

The cell autonomous regulation of T2Rs was originally found in the motile cilia of human airway epithelia (Shah et al., 2009). In this cellular location, bitter compounds elicit a dose-dependent increase in [Ca2+]i and consequently augment ciliary beat frequency (Fig. 2 A). The mechanism by which calcium influences ciliary beat frequency remains to be determined. Probably, calcium regulates the ciliary beat frequency directly or indirectly via a cyclic nucleotide-dependent manner (Salathe, 2007). Another cell-autonomous action occurs in airway smooth muscle, wherein bitter tastants dose dependently relax precontracted airways (Deshpande et al., 2010; Zhang et al., 2013). What remains debatable is how bitter tastants relax this smooth muscle. Deshpande et al. (2010) proposed that bitter tastants activate big conductance Ca2+-activated K+ (BK) channels and hyperpolarize the membrane, leading to relaxation (Fig. 2 B, left side). But by directly measuring BK channel currents, we and others found that bitter tastants do not activate these channels but instead inhibit them (Zhang et al., 2012; Wei et al., 2015). We recently discovered that the βγ subunits of gustducin are critical for bitter tastant–induced airway relaxation. These subunits can shut down L-type voltage-dependent Ca2+ channels and decrease [Ca2+]i (which is raised by bronchoconstrictors), leading to the relaxation (Fig. 2 B, right side; Zhang et al., 2013).

The cell-autonomous model of the T2R signaling cascade. (A) Bitter tastants increase cilia beat frequency in airway epithelium. (B) Bitter tastants relax precontracted airway smooth muscle cells. cGMP, cyclic guanosine monophosphate.

The paracrine role of T2Rs was first reported in a specialized small intestine enteroendocrine cell (EEC). Increased Ca2+ from the T2R activation leads to the release of a peptide hormone cholecystokinin (CCK), which acts either through CCK2 receptors in the neighboring enterocytes to promote multidrug resistance protein 1 (also known as ATP-binding cassette B1 [ABCB1]) to pump bitter tasting toxins out of the cells (Fig. 3 A, right side of the panel; Jeon et al., 2011) or through CCK1 receptors in sensory fibers of the vagal nerve that then transmit signals to the brain to control food intake (Fig. 3 A, left side; Cummings and Overduin, 2007). Solitary chemosensory cells (SCCs) from the nasal and vomeronasal cavity, or brush cells from the trachea in rodents, were found to release acetylcholine upon stimulation with bitter chemicals or bacterial signals. Acetylcholine then activates nicotinic acetylcholine receptors in the nearby sensory nerve fibers, which in turn decreases the breathing rate and closes the vomeronasal organ (VNO), or, alternatively, induces neurogenic inflammation in the nasal cavity (Fig. 3 B; Finger et al., 2003; Ogura et al., 2010; Tizzano et al., 2010; Krasteva et al., 2011; Saunders et al., 2014). A similar protective reflex in the bladder was also found in urethral brush cells (Fig. 3 B; Deckmann et al., 2014). Very recently, it was demonstrated that tuft cells in the gut orchestrate type 2 immunity to parasitic infection through the canonical GPCR taste receptor (T1R or T2R) cascade and also form a feedforward loop resulting in their own hyperplasia (Fig. 3 C; Gerbe et al., 2016; Howitt et al., 2016; von Moltke et al., 2016).

The paracrine model of the T2R signaling cascade. (A) In the gut, dietary toxins or bitter compounds from bacteria activate T2Rs in EECs to release the peptide hormone CCK, which acts through CKK2 receptors in the neighboring enterocytes to promote ABCB1 to pump bitter-tasting toxins out of the enterocytes (right). Alternatively, CCK released by EECs can also activate CCK1 receptors on sensory fibers of the vagus nerve to send signals to the brain to limit food intake (left). (B) The paracrine model also operates in mouse SCCs from the nasal organ or VNO and in brush cells from the trachea and bladder, where bitter compounds or N-acyl homoserine lactones, bacterial quorum-sensing molecules, activate bitter-taste signaling to release Ach, which in turn activates sensory fibers to (a) initiate a protective reflex, leading to a decrease in respiratory rate or an increase in bladder contraction; (b) close the VNO duct; or (c) induce neurogenic inflammation in the nasal cavity. (C) In tuft cells from the gut, parasites activate the canonical taste cascade and release IL-25, which in turn increases the number of ILC2s and boosts the secretion of type 2 immune cytokines IL-13 and IL-4; these cytokines subsequently promote the hyperplasia of tuft cells and goblet cells.

The endocrine mechanism of T2R signaling operates in tissues or cells in which T2R activation releases hormones that can be circulated via the bloodstream. Intestinal EECs release glucagonlike peptide 1 (GLP-1), which diffuses across the extracellular fluids to enter the circulation, and then stimulates the release of insulin from pancreatic β cells (Fig. 4; Dotson et al., 2008; Kim et al., 2014).

The endocrine model of the T2R signaling pathway in EECs. These cells secrete GLP-1, which diffuses across the extracellular fluids to enter the circulation, and in turn stimulate the release of insulin from pancreatic β-cells.

Physiological roles of extraoral T2Rs

Shortly after the finding that gustducin is a G protein that couples with taste receptors in taste cells of the tongue (McLaughlin et al., 1992), this G protein was detected in gut cells by Höfer et al. (1996), raising the possibility that cells outside the oral cavity may use taste receptors as chemosensors. Indeed, several years later, Wu et al. (2002) and Finger et al. (2003) found T2Rs in the epithelia of the gut and nasal cavities, respectively. To date, T2Rs and their signaling components have been detected in a large number of cells and tissues located outside the mouth. Moreover, activation of these receptors produces a diverse range of biological responses under normal conditions. In this section, we summarize the physiological functions that are likely mediated by these receptors.

Innate immunity

Many mammalian organs directly contact the exterior, and such organs include, but are not limited to, those in the respiratory, gastrointestinal, reproduction, and urinary systems. Because of this external nature, these organs are readily and constantly exposed to a vast number of bacteria, fungi, and viruses, along with their derived substances. Therefore, a fundamental challenge to these organs is how to avoid infection. Intensive research has revealed that several immune mechanisms collaborate to achieve this. Of these mechanisms, innate immunity is a rapid response that is paramount for avoiding infection at the early stage. The epithelial barrier is a major component of innate immunity, which prevents microbe entry or pathogen colonization either by speeding up mucociliary clearance by increasing ciliary beat frequency or by directly producing antiorganismal compounds (Chaplin, 2010; Pastorelli et al., 2013; Shaykhiev and Crystal, 2013; Amjadi et al., 2014). Accumulating evidence suggests that T2R-mediated signaling contributes much to the innate immunity in the epithelia of the organs that are connected to the external environment.

Hitherto, most of the studies related to bitter tastants 'role in innate immunity have been focused on the respiratory system. Various T2Rs are expressed in the ciliated epithelial cells of human and rodent airways. Compared with primary cilia, which act as a sensory organelle, motile cilia function to move mucus or particles out of the airway. Human ciliated airway cells express T2R4, T2R43, and T2R46, and their activation with bitter chemicals increases [Ca2+]i and ciliary beat frequency, accelerating the clearance of microorganisms and their derived products (Shah et al., 2009). Interestingly, T2R38 is expressed in the apical membrane and cilia of human sinus epithelium, and its activation by its agonist or by microbe-derived quorum-sensing molecules (e.g., acyl-homoserine lactones [AHLs]) generates nitric oxide, a potent bactericide (Lee et al., 2012). Additionally, nitric oxide speeds up ciliary beat frequency in the human sinus epithelium through the guanylyl cyclase and protein kinase G pathway (Salathe, 2007). This phenomenon is conserved in mice, although mice do not have a T2R38 orthologue. Moreover, the response to quorum-sensing molecules depends on the canonical taste signaling components PLCβ2 and TRPM5, but not α-gustducin, based on genetic and pharmacological evidence (Lee et al., 2014a). Quorum-sensing molecules are a class of chemical signals regulating the expression of microbial genes involved in the formation of biofilm (Nealson et al., 1970; Nealson and Hastings, 1979; Eberhard et al., 1981; Davies et al., 1998; Marx, 2014). Once their concentration becomes sufficiently high, a biofilm is formed to protect the bacteria from the host immune defense system (Nealson et al., 1970; Nealson and Hastings, 1979; Eberhard et al., 1981; Davies et al., 1998; Marx, 2014). In this context, it makes sense that mammals use T2Rs as a sensory part of their rapid innate immune system to prevent bacteria from forming the biofilm.

The SCC is another type of airway epithelium cell harboring both T2Rs and most taste transduction components; it comprises 1% of cells in the surface of the respiratory system (Workman et al., 2015). Finger et al. (2003) first identified T2R-expressing SCCs in the rodent nasal cavity, which also houses many elements of the bitter taste signaling pathway, including Gα-gustducin, PLCβ2, and TRPM5 (Finger et al., 2003; Gulbransen et al., 2008; Lin et al., 2008). Bitter compounds or AHLs cause mouse nasal SCCs to release the neurotransmitter acetylcholine, which in turn stimulates neighboring peptidergic nociceptive trigeminal fibers to secrete calcitonin gene-related peptide and substance P, resulting in the initiation of a neurogenic inflammation response to block bacterial invasion (Saunders et al., 2014). Alternatively, the activated trigeminal fibers can mediate a protective reflex to depress the respiratory rate, thus avoiding further inhalation of irritating substances or microbes (Fig. 3 B; Finger et al., 2003; Tizzano et al., 2010; Krasteva et al., 2011). Recently, choline acetyltransferase enhanced green fluorescent protein (eGFP)–positive (ChAT-eGFP+) SCCs in the mouse VNO were shown to regulate VNO duct accessibility (Ogura et al., 2010). In the mouse trachea, ChAT-eGFP+ chemosensory cells (called brush cells) can regulate the breathing rate by sensing the local chemical composition; this uses a mechanism similar to that used by nasal SCCs, mentioned above (Fig. 3 B; Finger et al., 2003; Tizzano et al., 2010; Krasteva et al., 2011, 2012a). More recently, a similar brush cell response (i.e., acetylcholine release) has also been demonstrated in the mouse urethral system (Deckmann et al., 2014). In this system, hazardous bitter compounds bind with T2Rs in the brush cells, releasing acetylcholine, which then activates nearby urethral sensory nerve fibers and stimulates detrusor muscle contraction (Fig. 3 B; Deckmann et al., 2014). Further investigation of microorganism-derived materials is necessary to determine whether such a reflex also occurs when microbes access the urethra.

In human sinonasal epithelia, SCCs express a set of denatonium-responsive T2Rs that are absent in T2R38-expressing sinonasal ciliated cells and underlie a role distinct from the T2R38-mediated nitric oxide response observed in the ciliated epithelial cells (see above; Lee et al., 2012, 2014a). Activation of these T2Rs in SCCs propagates a calcium wave to the surrounding cells through gap junctions, causing a robust secretion of broad-spectrum antimicrobial peptides and β-defensin. However, they exert no effect on ciliary beat frequency. Interestingly, these SCCs also express T1R2/3 sweet taste receptors, which negatively regulate the T2R response. In healthy individuals, sweet taste receptors activated by airway surface liquid glucose (~ 0.5 mM) suppress T2R-mediated antimicrobial peptide secretion. However, during microbial infection, T1R2/3 is deactivated as the interior bacteria reduce the glucose concentration by consuming it, consequently increasing T2R-mediated antimicrobial peptide release (Lee and Cohen, 2014; Lee et al., 2014b). Therefore, the two different defense systems mediated by ciliated epithelial T2Rs and SCC T2Rs work in concert to maintain human lower airway health.

The mammalian gut is colonized by microbiota, which comprises a collection of bacteria, archaea, viruses, fungi, and parasites (Sommer and Bäckhed, 2013). The single layer of gut epithelial cells orchestrates many ways to surveil the microbes (Peterson and Artis, 2014). Although the first extraoral cells found to express α-gustducin were tuft cells (also called brush cells) within the rat gastrointestinal tract (Höfer et al., 1996), the finding of T2Rs in gut epithelium took place several years later (Wu et al., 2002), and it was not until earlier this year that three different groups (Gerbe et al., 2016; Howitt et al., 2016; von Moltke et al., 2016) demonstrated that tuft cells harness taste transduction signaling to initiate type 2 immunity against pathogens often copresent with symbiotic microbes. In detail, tuft cells sense the parasite infection via canonical taste signaling and secrete IL-25, which increases the number of innate lymphoid cells (ILC2s) and their production of type 2 immune cytokines IL-4 and IL-13. Subsequently, these cytokines promote hyperplasia of tuft cells and goblet cells by facilitating intestinal stem cell differentiation (Fig. 3 C). However, which T2Rs or whether other taste receptors are involved in this process remains to be determined. It is reasonable to speculate that a mechanism similar to that which has been revealed in the SCCs or brush cells in the airway may be used to monitor microbiota in the gut.

Secretion

Endocrine, paracrine, and autocrine secretions are essential for maintaining body homeostasis. The gut is the largest endocrine organ and the source of gut hormones (Ahlman and Nilsson, 2001). Besides working as an innate defense barrier, intestinal epithelial cells house different subsets of cells that release hormones.

EECs, scattered along the epithelial layer of the GI tract from the stomach to the rectum, respond to an ingested meal by secreting a variety of gut hormones, including CCK, GLP-1, glucose-dependent insulinotropic peptide, peptide YY, somatostatin, ghrelin, and serotonin. These hormones perform functions ranging from modulating food intake to regulating insulin release (Psichas et al., 2015; Gribble and Reimann, 2016). The secretion from EECs is mainly triggered by the sensing of luminal contents via GPCRs, including the T2R family (Psichas et al., 2015). It is known that denatonium stimulates the mouse EEC cell line STC-1 to release CCK dose dependently, as does phenylthiocarbamide for GLP-1 (Wu et al., 2002; Chen et al., 2006). The extract of Hoodia gordonii activates T2R14 to secrete CCK in the human EEC line HuTu-80 (Le Nevé et al., 2010). Bitter tastants or extracts from bitter herbs cause GLP-1 secretion in the human EEC line NCI-H716 (Jang et al., 2007; Dotson et al., 2008; Suh et al., 2015).

In vivo studies also indicate that EECs have the capability to secrete hormones to regulate plasma glucose or the ingestion of toxic substances. Intragastric administration of bitter chemicals leads to a rise in the plasma ghrelin level, resulting in a short-term increase in food intake. This effect is subsequently followed by a long-term decrease in food intake caused by a delay in gastric emptying (Janssen et al., 2011). A gavage of denatonium followed by glucose or oral administration of herb extracts to db/db mice induces GLP-1 and subsequent insulin secretion, ultimately leading to a decrease in the blood glucose level (Kim et al., 2014; Suh et al., 2015). Nevertheless, in vivo direct evidence is needed to demonstrate that the glucose drop is exclusively caused by EECs because no immunostaining evidence exists depicting a colocalization between EEC markers and T2Rs, although α-gustducin and TRPM5 have both been detected in serotonin and GLP-1–producing ECCs.

In addition to EECs, SCCs in the gut also contain taste signaling elements. In the mouse stomach, α-gustducin–harboring SCCs locate in close proximity to the ghrelin and serotonin-releasing EECs. This has led to a hypothesis that SCCs perform a chemosensory role by forwarding messages from the lumen onto the EECs, which then secrete hormones (Hass et al., 2007). This seems possible, as denatonium causes an increase in Ca2+ in TRPM5-expressing SCCs, followed by a delayed Ca2+ response in the adjacent epithelium (Bezençon et al., 2008). However, T2R proteins have yet to be detected in gastrointestinal SCCs, although various T2R transcripts have been found in the epithelia of humans and rodents.

T2Rs also play secretion roles in the lower gastrointestinal tract.

T2R108 ligand 6-n-propyl-2-thiouracil (6-PTU) induces anion secretion in the human and rat large intestine, and this action is considered to be a protective response meant to flush out noxious irritants (Kaji et al., 2009). Hence, one function of T2Rs in the gastrointestinal epithelial cells is to limit the influence of toxic compounds by preventing their further intake or accelerating their excretion.

Several T2Rs are expressed in human and mouse thyrocytes and in human thyrocyte line Nthy-Ori3-1. These T2Rs negatively regulate thyroid-stimulating hormone-dependent iodide efflux in thyrocytes and thereby decrease the secretion of thyroid hormone. This might mediate a protective response to the ingestion of toxic compounds (Clark et al., 2015). Beyond these secretion roles in the gastrointestinal tract and thyroid, T2Rs in respiratory epithelium cells mediate the secretion of nitric oxide, neurotransmitters, and antimicrobial peptides (Krasteva et al., 2011; Lee et al., 2012, 2014b).

Contraction and relaxation

T2Rs in smooth muscles have attracted a lot of attention ever since Deshpande et al. (2010) reported that T2R agonists cause the relaxation of precontracted airway smooth muscle ex vivo and decrease airway resistance in vivo in mice. This relaxation is paradoxical, as bitter tastants can increase $[Ca2+]i$ (to the level induced by bronchoconstrictors) in human cultured airway smooth muscle cells (Deshpande et al., 2010) or to a more modest level in freshly isolated relaxed mouse airway smooth muscle cells (Zhang et al., 2013). This paradox has stimulated a wave of research into the underlying relaxation mechanisms. Results have been controversial. In addition to the two mechanisms described in the T2R signaling transductions section (Fig. 2 B), several other possibilities have been proposed for bitter tastants–induced relaxation of airway smooth muscle. Grassin-Delyle et al. (2013) suggested the involvement of the phosphatidylinositol-3 kinase (PI3K) pathway based on studies using intact human bronchi. Tan and Sanderson (2014) determined that bitter tastants directly inhibit InsP3R-mediated Ca2+ oscillations to relax airways. Tazzeo et al. (2012) proposed that bitter tastants (such as caffeine) may act downstream of myosin light chain kinase to interfere with the contractile apparatus, causing airway smooth muscle relaxation.

Although the cellular mechanisms are still debatable, a consensus is that bitter tastants are potentially potent bronchodilators, as they produce airway relaxation and protect against airway constriction in vivo better than some of the currently used asthma medicines. To date, a variety of bitter compounds have been found to relax precontracted airway smooth muscle from humans, mice, and guinea pigs (Deshpande et al., 2010; Pulkkinen et al., 2012; Zhang et al., 2013; Tan and Sanderson, 2014; Camoretti-Mercado et al., 2015). An attractive feature of using bitter tastants as bronchodilators is that these compounds can produce relaxation in airways precontracted by a broad spectrum of agonists (although there are some efficacy differences; Pulkkinen et al., 2012; Camoretti-Mercado et al., 2015). For example, in guinea pig trachea, denatonium selectively inhibits contractions induced by carbachol, whereas chloroquine uniformly inhibits contractions evoked by prostaglandin E(2), thromboxane receptor agonist U-46619, leukotriene D(4), histamine, and antigen (Pulkkinen et al., 2012); in human airways, chloroquine inhibits [Ca2+]i elevation and contractile responses normally induced by histamine, but not those induced by endothelin-1. Conversely, aristolochic acid prevents contractile responses induced by endothelin-1, but not those induced by histamine (Camoretti-Mercado et al., 2015). This necessitates studying how each bitter compound performs against different bronchoconstrictors to appropriately assess its effectiveness as a bronchodilator.

Several studies have demonstrated the roles of bitter compounds in regulating vascular smooth muscle contractility. Manson et al. (2014) reported that bitter ligands for human T2R3, 4, 10, and 14 induce relaxation of precontracted human pulmonary arteries, guinea pig aorta, and mouse aorta. This relaxation is independent of the inhibition of L-type Ca2+ channels or activation of

BK channels but is dependent on the formation of caveolae (Manson et al., 2014). Lund et al. (2013) revealed that hT2R46 is expressed in human aorta vascular smooth muscle cells, and intravenous injection of denatonium via catheter in rats leads to a transient drop in blood pressure. Interestingly, Upadhyaya et al. (2014) reported that dextromethorphan induces a vasoconstriction via a T2R1-mediated Ca2+ response in human pulmonary artery smooth muscle. The authors proposed that the calcium increase from the canonical T2R signaling pathway directly activates myosin light chain kinase and subsequently increases the phosphorylated myosin light chain, leading to constriction (Upadhyaya et al., 2014).

T2Rs and taste signaling elements are also present in mouse and human gastrointestinal smooth muscle cells. Bitter tastants induce a contraction when applied at lower concentrations (e.g., <100 μM for denatonium) and a relaxation at higher concentrations (e.g., >500 μM for denatonium). Intragastric administration of denatonium leads to a T2R-dependent delay in gastric emptying. Moreover, after intragastric denatonium administration, healthy volunteers showed an impaired fundic relaxation in response to nutrient infusion and a decreased nutrient volume tolerance and increased satiation during an oral nutrient challenge test (Avau et al., 2015). As the role of T2Rs in the gastrointestinal epithelia cannot be ruled out in these in vivo experiments, these results might be influenced by both epithelia and smooth muscle in the gastrointestinal tract. Undoubtedly, the protective role of T2Rs makes them valuable targets for drug development to treat gastrointestinal motility diseases.

Foster et al. (2013) reported that cardiac myocytes express five T2Rs and their downstream signaling elements. Using a heterologous expression system, Foster et al. (2014a) de-orphaned three of the five T2Rs expressed in these cells. In their function study, the authors found that sodium thiocyanate, a T2R108 agonist, elicited a 30–40% decrease in left ventricular pressure and systolic pressure, as well as a steady increase in aortic pressure, whereas sodium benzoate, a T2R137 agonist, and sodium arbutin, a T2R143 agonist, displayed a minor or modest effect, respectively, on these cardiac functions (Orsmark-Pietras et al., 2013; Foster et al., 2014a). Moreover, these effects are abrogated by Gi and Gβγ inhibitors (e.g., pertussis toxin and gallein). Therefore, T2R signaling may play an important role in regulating cardiac functions.

Reproduction and urination

T2Rs in the genitourinary system has been another area of attention. T2Rs and taste transduction cascade components (α-gustducin, Gγ13, and PLCCβ2) have been detected in different stages of spermatogenesis (with TRPM5 being observed only in the later spermatid phase; Li and Zhou, 2012). Bitter chemicals induce a rise in [Ca2+]i in spermatids, and individual spermatids exhibit different ligand activation profiles, indicating a unique T2R profile in each spermatid (Xu et al., 2013). Moreover, depletion of T2R105 results in smaller testes and is sufficient to lead to male infertility (Li and Zhou, 2012). These results suggest a crucial role for T2R receptors in spermatogenesis and a possible function in sensing and avoiding noxious chemicals that are present during fertilization.

In the female reproductive system, human T2R38 is expressed in the amniotic epithelium, syncytiotrophoblast, and decidua cells in human placenta, and in a placental cell line (JEG-3; Wölfle et al., 2016). Although the T2R38 agonist diphenidol evokes calcium influx in the placental cell line, there is no further functional characterization of T2R38 in placenta (Wölfle et al., 2016).

Seven T2Rs and α-gustducin are expressed in mouse whole kidney (Rajkumar et al., 2014; Liu et al., 2015). Conditional ablation of T2R105-positive cells causes an increase in the size of the glomerulus and renal tubule, accompanied by a lower cell density in the glomerulus (Liu et al., 2015). These results suggest an essential role of T2R105 in maintaining the structure and consequent homeostasis in bodily fluids and electrolytes (Liu et al., 2015).

As mentioned previously, activation of T2Rs in urethral chemosensory cells initiates a reflex loop, leading to bladder contraction (Deckmann et al., 2014). In this context, it is interesting that Zhai et al. (2016) showed that human and mouse detrusor smooth muscle express T2Rs, and T2R agonists can directly relax precontracted detrusor muscle strips. In vivo study showed that oral gavage of the bitter compound chloroquine suppresses overactive bladder symptoms in mice that possess partial bladder outlet obstruction. Thus, T2Rs are potential targets for treating this disorder.

Therefore, T2Rs appear to have a versatile modulatory role in reproduction and urination; however, unlike in other systems, their roles remain largely to be determined.

Other roles

Many T2R transcripts have been detected in polymorphonuclear neutrophils. Knockdown of highly abundant T2R43 or T2R31 in these cells remarkably blocks the chemotactic trans-migration induced by saccharin (Malki et al., 2015). Another study showed that human neutrophils express T2R38, and its binding with quorum-sensing molecules (N-(3-oxododecanoyl)-l-homoserinelactone or AHL-12) induces migration of neutrophils (Maurer et al., 2015). Additionally, a recent investigation showed that phagocytes also express T2R38, which can be activated by AHL-12 (Gaida et al., 2016a). These results suggest that bitter tastants function within the immune system by binding to food-borne substances that enter the bloodstream after ingestion, molecules produced by bacterial infections, or harmful endogenous metabolites.

Several investigations have demonstrated the existence of T2Rs in the different compartments of the central nervous system, such as the brain stem, brain cells, parabrachial nucleus, and horoid plexus (Singh et al., 2011; Dehkordi et al., 2012; Tomás et al., 2016). Although some bitter chemicals have the capability to cross the brain–blood barrier, it remains to be determined whether their concentrations could reach the high micromolar level that is needed to activate many T2Rs. It would be interesting to find out whether, within the central nervous system, there are endogenous bitter-tasting compounds that can be highly effectively at activating T2Rs. If so, T2Rs in the central nervous system could serve as sensors for these ligands.

T2Rs have also been detected in several other tissues or organs. Several T2Rs have been detected in human skin biopsies and in the immortal keratinocyte cell line; bitter compounds (diphenidol and amarogentin) induce the expression of differentiation markers in human skin primary cells (Wölfle et al., 2015). T2Rs and taste transduction pathway components are expressed in the ChAT-eGFP+ brush cells in the murine auditory tube, submucosal glands of the larynx and trachea, and the thymic medulla, and they may function as sensors for the composition of the local microenvironment, as has been demonstrated for SCCs and brush cells in the airway (Krasteva et al., 2012b; Panneck et al., 2014; Krasteva-Christ et al., 2015). However, direct experiments are needed to confirm this.

Potential roles of extraoral T2Rs in disease

Several studies have begun to reveal that T2R mutants can cause or contribute to diseases in the extraoral tissues, highlighting the important roles that these receptors play under pathophysiological conditions. T2R genes do not contain introns in their protein-coding regions, and their expression levels are usually low under normal conditions. These characteristics may lead to changes in their expression level under different pathological conditions. In this section, we summarize both T2R mutations and/or changes in T2R expression level that occur in various diseases and disorders. The major T2Rs and their associated disorders and diseases are listed in Table 1.

Table 1.

T2R-associated disorders and diseases

Open in a separate window

T2R polymorphisms

T2R polymorphisms dictate taste preference and extraoral T2R-mediated pathophysiology. Several excellent studies and reviews have summarized changes in bitter taste caused by T2R genetic variants and polymorphisms (Kim et al., 2003; Bufe et al., 2005; Li et al., 2011; Campa et al., 2012; Keller et al., 2013; Risso et al., 2014). In this section, we focus on the alteration in extraoral function attributed to T2R polymorphisms. Of all T2R family members, T2R38 polymorphism is the most extensively investigated one. The T2R38 protein has two common variants that differ in the amino acid residues at positions 49, 262, and 296. The functional variant contains proline, alanine, and valine, respectively, in these positions, so the genotype is designated as PAV, whereas the nonfunctional form contains alanine, valine, and isoleucine to give rise to the AVI genotype. Therefore, the combination of these two variants generates three common genotypes, i.e., two homozygotes, PAV/PAV and AVI/AVI, and one heterozygote, PAV/AVI. Most of the work on the relationship between T2R38 polymorphisms and respiratory disease has been published by Cohen and his colleagues. These authors showed that the functional T2R38 PAV/PAV phenotype has a much lower infection rate from gram-negative bacteria than the other two genotypes (Lee and Cohen, 2013). The same group further showed that nonfunctional T2R38 genotypes (AVI/AVI and AVI/PAV) are present in >90% of the chronic rhinosinusitis population undergoing functional endoscopic sinus surgery (Adappa et al., 2014). They also found that homozygous ΔF508 cystic fibrosis patients with nonfunctional alleles exhibit more severe sinonasal symptoms (Adappa et al., 2016b). Finally, they determined that individuals with T2R38 functional homozygotes have more than a threefold improvement in surgical outcomes when compared with chronic rhinosinusitis patients possessing nonfunctional homozygotes or heterozygotes (Adappa et al., 2016a). Most recently, they found that among 59 chronic rhinosinusitis patients, an inverse linear association exists between in vitro biofilm formation and phenylthiocarbamide taste intensity ratings (P = 0.019; Adappa et al., 2016c). All of these results indicate that the T2R38 genotype is correlated with susceptibility, severity, and prognosis in upper respiratory disorders. However, a recent study on an Italian population showed that there is no association between T2R38 alleles and chronic rhinosinusitis

(Gallo et al., 2016). To firmly establish the role of T2R38 in chronic rhinosinusitis pathogenesis, studies with larger cohorts may be needed.

T2R38 polymorphism also relates to other diseases, such as cancer and cavities. Carrai et al. (2011) demonstrated that the nonfunctional group has an increased risk of colorectal cancer in comparison to the functional group in a population of Caucasian origin. In their study of the effect of T2R38 polymorphism on oral innate immunity, Gil et al. (2015) found a complicated set of responses when teeth were exposed to different pathogenic bacteria. In response to the cariogenic bacteria Streptococcus mutans, the transcription level of T2R38 in gingival epithelial cells was increased 4.3-fold in individuals with the PAV/PAV genotype, in contrast to a 1.2-fold increase in AVI/AVI individuals. IL-1α secretion in the PAV/PAV genotype was highest among all three genotypes, whereas the secretion of hBD-2 (antimicrobial peptide) and IL-1α in this genotype was decreased by 77% and 50%, respectively, after application of T2R38-specific small interfering RNA. When stimulated with the periodonatal pathogen Porphyromonas gingivalis, only the AVI/AVI T2R38 transcription levels increased by 4.4-fold. In addition, the levels of IL-1α and IL-8 were remarkably decreased when T2R38 was silenced (Gil et al., 2015). All these data suggest a genotype-dependent role of T2R38 in gingival innate immunity and a T2R38-associated risk of dental caries (Wendell et al., 2010) that may be more important than dietary habits.

Several other T2R polymorphisms are also correlated with various disorders as revealed by association studies. Dotson et al. (2008) found that the T2R19 haplotype is associated with altered glucose and insulin homeostasis. In a study involving 4,522 individuals aged 65 or above, Shiffman et al. (2008) reported that several human T2R50 single-nucleotide polymorphisms (SNPs; ID rs1376251) have strong associations with cardiovascular disease. Given that T2R50 is expressed in the heart (Foster et al., 2013), these SNPs may play a direct role in causing cardiovascular disease, rather than being involved in this disease indirectly via changes in food preference and diet, as proposed by Shiffman et al. (2008). Interestingly, another study indicated that the same SNPs of T2R50 could be useful in predicting statin-induced cardiovascular risk reduction in elderly women, but not in men (Akao et al., 2012); however, this sex difference disappeared when corrected for multiple comparisons (Akao et al., 2012). Thyroid-expressed T2R42 SNP (SNP type L196F) is associated with differences in circulating levels of thyroid hormones (Clark et al., 2015). Polymorphism of the position 212 bp upstream of human T2R16 is significantly associated with longevity—the frequency of A/A homozygotes is increased in older people. This site is most likely located in the promoter region for T2R16, suggesting a critical regulation role (Campa et al., 2012). Along with the important extraoral T2R functions, more T2R polymorphisms and their association with human health are expected to be discovered.

T2Rs in disorders and diseases

As airway smooth muscles express T2Rs and bitter compounds can profoundly relax constriction and decrease airway resistance in animal models of asthma, two questions immediately emerge: are T2R expression levels changed in asthmatic patients and are T2Rs desensitized in asthmatics, as are other GPCRs? Robinett et al. (2014) demonstrated that the mRNA expression levels of T2R10, 14, and 31 are not different between asthmatics and nonasthma controls, and T2R agonists relax airways from healthy and asthmatic specimens equally. As to the T2R desensitization, the same group found that pretreatment of human airway smooth muscle cells with a prototypical T2R agonist, quinine, results in ~30% desensitization in both [Ca2+]i response and airway relaxation (Robinett et al., 2011). However, there is no cross-desensitization between T2R and β2 adrenergic receptor–mediated relaxation (An et al., 2012), indicating that both therapies could be combined to treat asthma. In addition, several T2Rs are up-regulated in leukocytes in severe asthma patients, and T2R agonists can inhibit the release of proinflammatory cytokines and eicosanoid release from blood leukocytes

(Orsmark-Pietras et al., 2013). These findings suggest that T2R agonists may directly act on immune cells to perform their antiinflammatory role. All these findings underscore the potential of T2Rs as attractive targets for asthma management.

Although the pathophysiological roles of T2Rs have traditionally focused on the respiratory tract, their roles in other systems have begun to emerge. Low-fat diet or sterol depletion culture leads to an increase in the expression of most T2Rs in the mouse proximal intestine or the STC-1 cell line (a type of gut ECC), which may in turn stimulate the secretion of GLP-1 and CCK (Jeon et al., 2008). In human colonic mucosa, the number of T2R38 immunoreactive cells is significantly increased in overweight and obese subjects versus lean subjects and is also significantly correlated with body mass index values (Latorre et al., 2016). In the heart, the expression of T2R126, T2R135, and T2R143 is increased two- to threefold under starvation conditions both in vitro and in vivo (Foster et al., 2013). Subcutaneous administration of nitroglycerin (a myocardial antiischemic chemical) dramatically increases the T2R119 expression in heart and aorta (Csont et al., 2015). In the brains of Parkinson's disease patients, T2R5 and T2R50 are decreased, whereas T2R10 and T2R13 are augmented at both premotor and parkinsonian stages in the frontal cortex area (Garcia-Esparcia et al., 2013). Interestingly, T2R4, T2R5, T2R14, and T2R50 are down-regulated in the dorsolateral prefrontal cortex of schizophrenia patients (Ansoleaga et al., 2015). As the heart is not directly exposed to the external environment and the brain is further isolated by the blood–brain barrier, the changes in T2Rs in these systems raise the possibility that endogenous ligands for T2Rs exist throughout the human body.

T2R expression has also been detected in tumor or cancer cells. Singh et al. (2014) found that the expression of T2R4 is down-regulated in breast cancer cells compared with noncancerous mammary epithelial cells, suggesting a mechanism by which the breast cancer cells may escape from apoptosis, which would otherwise be induced by bitter compounds. In a study of pancreatic cancer, Gaida et al. (2016a) found that T2R38 is expressed in both tumor cells from pancreatic cancer patients and tumor-derived cell lines. Moreover, the T2R38-specific ligand phenylthiourea or natural ligand AHL-12 activate mitogen-activated protein kinases p38 and ERK1/2 and up-regulate NFATc1 in a G protein–dependent manner. Intriguingly, although there is no correlation between the frequency of T2R38-positive tumor cells and clinical and pathological parameters, the T2R38 ligands increase the expression of efflux transporter ABCB1, suggesting the possible engagement of T2R38 in the chemoresistance of pancreatic cancer (Gaida et al., 2016b).

Future perspectives

Recent advances have discovered the widespread extent of extraoral T2Rs unearthed the important roles these receptors play in a variety of cellular functions, and have shown that their pathologies may potentially contribute to several disease conditions. At the same time, studies have raised many important questions about these receptors and have uncovered several challenges that need to be overcome to further deepen our understanding of extraoral T2R biology.

Profiling T2R expression

Owing to the lack of well-documented antibodies for T2Rs (in particular for mouse T2Rs), the expression profiling of T2Rs in the extraoral tissues has been largely generated using in situ hybridization with antisense probes to T2Rs (Foster et al., 2013; Prandi et al., 2013) or quantitative real-time PCR or reverse transcript PCR with a template (but without transcriptase as a control to confirm no genome DNA contamination; Shah et al., 2009; Deshpande et al., 2010; Foster et al., 2013; Xu et al., 2013; Zhang et al., 2013; Deckmann et al., 2014). As to the first method, not every laboratory can satisfy its technical requirements. With regard to the latter two, the ways to eliminate genome DNA involve purification of mRNA with poly(T)-tag (Raz et al., 2011), digestion by DNase (Raz et al., 2011), or filtering by a genome-specific binding column. Most studies use DNA digestion or a DNA-binding column, even though the current commonly used DNases or filters cannot completely remove genome contamination. This shortcoming could result in trace contamination with genome DNA in the samples; additionally, it casts doubts on the T2R expression profile because T2R genes are intronless (Cui et al., 2007) and the expression level of T2Rs in extraoral tissues is very low, therefore requiring a large number of PCR cycles for quantification (Clark et al., 2012). Interestingly, the DNase for eliminating genome DNA in RNA sequencing can yield higher-quality RNA preparations. Utilization of this DNase for T2R expression could generate more reliable results. However, generating specific antibodies against T2Rs to visualize these receptors in cells and tissues could provide a more accurate estimate of T2R expression levels and their cellular location. This in turn could provide insight into the potential roles of T2Rs in different cells and tissues.

De-orphaning nonhuman T2Rs

Although most human T2Rs are de-orphaned, the majority of T2Rs in other species are orphan receptors (Meyerhof et al., 2010; Ji et al., 2014). Identification of agonists and antagonists for T2Rs would facilitate the study of the physiological roles of T2Rs. One method to determine ligands of T2Rs is to isolate cells that express known T2R(s) and their signaling components and stimulate them with different bitter compounds. Gulbransen et al. (2008) was the first to use this approach to demonstrate that the bitter compound denatonium could activate T2R108 in the SCCs; this was determined by examining the Ca2+ response in either Trmp5-GFP+ or gustducin-GFP+ isolated nasal SCCs (Chandrashekar et al., 2000; Finger et al., 2003). This approach is applicable to cells that express only one or a few T2Rs, and it would be less useful for cell types that express multiple T2Rs. A more general approach to de-orphaning T2Rs is to engineer a T2R signaling system in heterologous expression cells, often HEK293 cells. For human T2R expression, T2Rs fused with cell membrane–targeting peptides coexpress with a chimeric Gα16–gust44 and, in some cases, transport protein 3 (RTP3) or RTP4 to enhance the transport of T2Rs to the cell membrane (Ueda et al., 2003; Behrens et al., 2006; Deshpande et al., 2010; Ji et al., 2014). Ilegems et al. (2010) also demonstrated that receptor expression enhanced protein 2 boosts the responsiveness of human T2R16 and T2R44 to their ligands. It would be interesting to determine whether a similar expression strategy would work for T2Rs from other species.

Receptor antagonists can help dissect receptor function. To date, a handful of T2R antagonists from different sources (primarily from plants) have been found. Similar to T2R agonists (Meyerhof et al., 2010; Levit et al., 2014), T2R antagonists may interact with one T2R or multiple T2Rs. Likewise, a single T2R might be inactivated by more than one antagonist. Probenecid, an Food and Drug Administration–approved inhibitor of the multidrug resistance protein 1 transporter and used to treat gout in clinics, inhibits human T2R16, T2R38, and T2R43, but not T2R31 (Greene et al., 2011) and has been successfully applied to probe T2R's physiological roles (Pydi et al., 2015). GIV3727, an inhibitor of the human sweet taste receptor, inhibits T2R31 and T2R43 (Slack et al., 2010). Sakuranetin, 6-methoxysakuranetin, and jaceosidin, isolated from the leaves of the native North American plant Eriodictyon californicum, are T2R31 antagonists. Derived from edible plants, 3β-hydroxypelenolide or 3β-hydroxydihydrocostunolide can inhibit several T2Rs with different sensitivity (Brockhoff et al., 2011). Pydi et al. (2014, 2015) identified two amino acid derivatives, γ-aminobutryic acid and Nα, Nα-Bis(carboxymethyl)-l-lysine, and a plant hormone abscisic acid as competitive inhibitors of quinine-activated T2R4. Recently, three flavones (i.e., 4'-fluoro-6-methoxyflavanone, 6,3'-dimethoxyflavanone, and 6-methoxyflavanone) have been demonstrated to inhibit T2R39, and 6-methoxyflavanone also inhibits T2R14 (Roland et al., 2014). These antagonists should be useful to probe the physiological roles of human T2Rs expressed in different extraoral cells and tissues. But the number of known antagonists and the number of T2Rs they act on are very limited; further exploration is needed.

Analyzing extraoral T2R functions genetically

Besides the expression profiling of T2Rs, the roles of T2Rs in extraoral tissues in humans have been studied by using T2R agonists and antagonists and the inhibitors of T2R signaling components. These approaches have been applied to mice, although occasionally genetic deletion of T2R signaling components such as α-gustducin (Janssen et al., 2011; Lee et al., 2014a; Avau et al., 2015) and TRMP5 (Lee et al., 2014a; Saunders et al., 2014) have been used. To dissect the roles of T2Rs, a desirable approach is to genetically ablate these receptors. So far, only T2R105 (Li and Zhou, 2012; Rajkumar et al., 2014) and T2R131 (Voigt et al., 2012, 2015; Prandi et al., 2013; Soultanova et al., 2015) have been studied genetically to some extent. A potential challenge when probing T2R function with genetic approaches is that T2Rs may be redundant (as many T2R agonists activate multiple T2R receptors); therefore, deletion of a single T2R may have little effect. However, the fact that a cell type or tissue may express only a small subset of T2Rs, e.g., five in rodent heart (Foster et al., 2013), offers opportunities to knock out the entire subset of T2Rs using newly developed, highly efficient genomic editing methods such as CRISPR/Cas9 technology. Most T2Rs locate in genomes in just a few clusters, making it easier to knock out all the T2Rs in mice or other species with this technology after a few cycles of cross-breeding (Wang et al., 2013; Foster et al., 2014b). It is expected that these T2R transgenic knockout mice will greatly facilitate our understanding of the physiological roles of T2Rs in the extraoral systems.

Identifying physiological ligands for T2Rs

Canonically, T2Rs are known to detect bitter tastants in the diet. With recent advances in understanding the role of oral microbiota (Avila et al., 2009; Dewhirst et al., 2010), it is reasonable to speculate that T2Rs may also sense symbiotic microorganisms and their derivatives in the oral cavity. The same idea could be also applied to the T2Rs in the organs, which directly contact external environments. In other words, T2Rs in gastroenterological and respiratory systems could function as sensors of bitter tastants that are injected or inhaled, and also of microorganisms and their derivatives. However, because the threshold for T2R activation is high, generally in the micromolar range, it is not clear what would be the primary or physiological ligands for T2Rs in the systems that do not directly interact with the external environment. One possibility is that certain bitter-tasting endogenous bioactive compounds that circulate in the bloodstream may serve as physiological ligands for T2Rs in the extraoral cells and tissues. Interestingly, using a heterologous expression system, Lossow et al. (2016) recently reported that progesterone can activate mouse T2R110 and T2R114, raising the possibility that this reproductively important hormone may be one of the endogenous ligands for T2Rs. The method by which Yoshikawa et al. (2013) identified a physiological ligand for olfactory receptor 288 using fractionation of crude tissue extracts may be instructive for searching for T2Rs 'endogenous ligands.

Studying T2R transcription regulation

So far, only one regulator, sterol regulatory element–binding protein (SREBP-2), has been demonstrated to target the transcription machinery of T2Rs. SREBP-2 activates the transcription of T2R138 by directly binding to the promoter region in STC-1 cells (Jeon et al., 2008). Studying T2R regulators would facilitate identifying T2R physiological functions, especially when T2R knockout mice are lacking. T2Rs locate in chromosomes as clusters, suggesting that common gene regulatory mechanisms may exist to control the T2R loci. For example, after analyzing regions near T2R loci in silico, Foster et al. (2013, 2014a, 2015) detected cis-regulatory domains, which are overlaps of histone marks and DNase-I hypersensitivity regions and indicative of active enhancer and promoter regions, in the mouse T2R143/135/126 cluster as well as in the regions proximal to human T2R5 and T2R14 loci. Besides such local control regions, long-range cis-regulatory elements in chromatin may also exist to regulate T2R transcription; these elements, despite a large separation along the DNA, can interact with each other to work in a regulatory capacity because of their proximity in 3-D (Harmston and Lenhard, 2013; Heinz et al., 2015). A detailed analysis of the transcript regulatory elements of T2Rs would be informative to enhance our understanding of T2Rs' roles.

Conclusion

Cumulative evidence indicates that T2Rs mediate a variety of functions in nonlingual tissues and may underlie several human diseases or disorders. Targeting of T2Rs in extraoral tissues is showing promise for the development of new therapeutics. The wide expression of extraoral T2Rs underscores the possibility that they might be accountable for the many side effects of current medicines because most drugs have a bitter taste (Clark et al., 2012). However, all this reinforces the necessity to fully characterize T2R physiology and pathophysiology at different extraoral locations. With this knowledge, we may one day understand the true biological basis through which bitter drugs can act as "good medicine."

A Bitter Taste in Your Heart

Conor J. Bloxham,1 Simon R. Foster,2 and Walter G. Thomas1,*
Author information Article notes Copyright and License information PMC Disclaimer

Go to:

Abstract

The human genome contains ~ 29 bitter taste receptors (T2Rs), which are responsible for detecting thousands of bitter ligands, including toxic and aversive compounds. This sentinel function varies between individuals and is underpinned by naturally occurring T2R polymorphisms, which have also been associated with disease. Recent studies have reported the expression of T2Rs and their downstream signaling components within non-gustatory tissues, including the heart. Though the precise role of T2Rs in the heart remains unclear, evidence points toward a role in cardiac contractility and overall vascular tone. In this review, we summarize the extra-oral expression of T2Rs, focusing on evidence for expression in heart; we speculate on the range of potential ligands that may activate them; we define the possible signaling pathways they activate; and we argue that their discovery in heart predicts an, as yet, unappreciated cardiac physiology.

Keywords: taste receptors, G protein-coupled receptors, cardiac physiology, signaling, polymorphisms, bitter ligands

Go to:

Extra-Oral Expression of Bitter T2Rs

TAS2R/T2Rs (gene and protein) were first discovered within type II taste receptor cells in the tongue and act as sentinels in protecting against the ingestion of potentially toxic substances (Chandrashekar et al., 2000; Lu et al., 2017). Since these pioneering studies, T2R expression has been reported in a multitude of extra-oral tissues, including the gut, lungs, brain, and heart (Shah et al., 2009; Foster et al., 2013; Garcia-Esparcia et al., 2013), but their complete function(s) in physiology and pathophysiology remain to be defined. In Table 1, we have summarized the location, expression profile and proposed function for the T2R family across a range of human tissues and cells. In regard to function, we would offer a note of caution that a number of studies (listed in Table 1) have proposed functions based on stimulation with various bitter compounds in the micromolar to millimolar range where the selectivity and specificity toward T2Rs may reasonably be questioned. Despite this, the expression of T2Rs within the cardiovascular system, particularly the heart and vasculature, has gained significant interest in recent years. Following our initial discovery of TAS2Rs within the heart (Foster et al., 2013), a number of subsequent studies have focused on the vasculature (Lund et al.,

2013; Manson et al., 2014; Upadhyaya et al., 2014; Chen et al., 2017). An unambiguous definition of their function has, however, lagged behind the capacity to demonstrate their expression.

TABLE 1

Distribution, expression profile, proposed function, and technique used for the detection of extra-oral TAS2R/T2R expression.

Open in a separate window

The expression of TAS2Rs in different tissues and cell lines has been examined using RT-PCR, qPCR, microarray techniques as well as RNAseq (Flegel et al., 2013). Most recently, Jaggupilli et al. (2017) used nCounter gene expression analysis to characterize the expression of the 29 human TAS2Rs in a variety of cell lines (Table 1). Their results showed that TAS2R14 and TAS2R20 were highly expressed; TAS2R3, −4, −5, −10, −13, −19, and −50 were moderately expressed; TAS2R8, −9, −21 and −60 had low level of expression; and TAS2R7, −16, −38, −39, −40, −41, and −42 were barely detectable. The nCounter technique relies on hybridization of complementary probes (spanning 100 nucleotide bases) for each gene, and hence, TAS2R30, −31, −43, −45, and −46 could not be accurately discerned from one another, as they share >92% homology. Nevertheless, this data clearly shows that some T2Rs are broadly and differentially expressed, whereas others are more restricted in their tissue distribution.

Go to:

Model Systems for Expressing T2Rs and Defining Their Function

In attempting to define the function of, and to identify ligands for, the T2Rs, researchers have established heterologous expression systems in human cells (e.g., HEK293 or HEK293T) (Meyerhof et al., 2010). However, the use of these cells for understanding the underlying mechanisms and signaling pathways within cardiovascular tissues/cells has obvious limitations. Firstly, due to the insufficient cell surface targeting of T2Rs in heterologous cells (Chandrashekar et al., 2000), chimeric T2Rs encompassing the amino terminus of the rat somatostatin receptor subtype 3 are often used to improve expression and functionality (Bufe et al., 2002; Behrens et al., 2006). Furthermore, a chimeric G protein consisting of the Gα16 and 44 amino acids of gustducin attached to the carboxyl terminus is widely used in calcium mobilization assays (Liu et al., 2003; Ueda et al., 2003). Gα16 has been coined the 'universal adaptor' due to its ability to interact with numerous GPCRs and provides a robust readout for receptor activation, including for T2Rs (Ueda et al., 2003). While these artificial heterologous systems have proven useful in identifying ligands for orphan receptors (Meyerhof et al., 2010) and interrogating the structure-function aspects of T2Rs (Brockhoff et al., 2010), the field is now moving toward more relevant cellular models with endogenous receptors and signaling partners (Freund et al., 2018).

Studies using the aforementioned heterologous expression system have demonstrated that the majority of T2Rs form oligomers, both homodimers and heterodimers (Kuhn et al., 2010). However, unlike the situation for umami/sweet taste sensation (requiring dimerization of T1R1/T1R2 and T1R1/T1R3), T2R homodimers did not appear to alter the pharmacology of the receptors, nor do they have obvious influence on protein expression or membrane localization (Kuhn et al., 2010). In contrast, Kim et al. (2016) used immuno-fluorescent microscopy to show that the co-expression of the adrenergic (ADRβ2) receptor with T2R14 resulted in a ~ 3-fold increase in cell-surface expression of T2R14. Co-immunoprecipitation and biomolecular fluorescence complementation experiments confirmed that the increase of cell-surface expression was attributed to the formation of T2R14:ADRβ2 heterodimers. These complexes may be particularly important in heart where the actions of adrenergic receptors are well described. Interestingly, co-immunoprecipitation and co-internalization of ADRβ2:M71 OR (mouse 71 olfactory receptor) was observed in response to their specific ligands (Hague et al., 2004). These seminal observations in heterologous systems need to be confirmed and extended with endogenous models to clarify our understanding of how T2Rs function in vivo and to define their potential modulation of (or by) established GPCRs.

Another important issue in considering model expression systems for studying T2Rs is the requirement for appropriate accessory proteins and correct post-translational processing. It is now well-established that chemosensory receptors [e.g., odorant (McClintock et al., 1997) and pheromone (Loconto et al., 2003) receptors] rely on endogenous proteins in order to be targeted to the cell-surface. A study by Behrens et al. (2006) demonstrated that certain members of the receptor-transporting protein (RTP) and receptor expression enhancing protein (REEP) families enhance cell-surface localization and functionality of certain TAS2Rs, likely through protein–protein interactions. Furthermore, it was shown that varying combinations of these proteins are expressed endogenously within tissues (circumvallate papillae and testis) that express TAS2R genes. Interestingly, the human heart differentially expresses REEP 1, 2, 3, 5, and 6 across heart regions (Doll et al., 2017), suggesting that efficient cell-surface TAS2R expression may also be region specific. Nonetheless, these trafficking proteins do not universally promote T2R functionality, for instance T2R14 showed no increase in capacity to mobilize calcium when co-expressed with either RTP or REEP (Behrens et al., 2006). There is accumulating evidence that the degree of T2R membrane insertion is dependent on the specific tissue. As T2Rs are detected in a myriad of tissues, multiple endogenous mechanisms may contribute to their appropriate expression and localization. As for many GPCRs, N-glycosylation of T2Rs is important for cell-surface localization–Reichling et al. (2008) reported that glycosylation of the second extracellular loop is essential for the recruitment (via association with the cellular chaperone calnexin) and insertion of TAS2Rs in the cell membrane; moreover, the function of non-glycosylated TAS2R16 could be rescued when co-expressed with RTP3 and RTP4.

Go to:

The Cardiac Gpcr Repertoire Includes T2Rs

The human heart expresses over 200 different GPCRs (Wang et al., 2018), some of which are critical for regulating cardiac morphology and function (Capote et al., 2015). Intriguingly, the gene transcripts for more than half of the TAS2R family were detected in both left ventricle and right atria (Foster et al., 2013) ranging in abundance between that observed for two classically important cardiac GPCRs – the angiotensin II type 1 receptor and β1-adrenergic receptor (ADRβ1). It is notable that the expression of TAS2R14 was equivalent to that of ADRβ1 in the left ventricle. These findings are supported by publicly available Illumina Human BodyMap 2.0 project RNA-seq dataset (Flegel et al., 2013), which showed widespread TAS2R expression in human tissues and highest expression of TAS2R14 in heart. It is important, however, to note that T2Rs are not uniformly detected by all techniques, with TAS2R9, TAS2R39, and TAS2R45 not detected in the Illumina RNA-seq data set, but detected by qPCR (Foster et al., 2013). These differences could reflect individual variations, noting the body map is from one patient or the more specific nature of RNA-seq over qPCR. Interestingly, the expression of TAS2Rs are differentially regulated with age in mice (Foster et al., 2013), but not with sex or in heart failure (Foster et al., 2015a). Furthermore, analysis of the publicly available GTEx LDACC and BioGPS Human Cell Type and Tissue Gene Expression Profiles RNA-seq datasets, highlight the expression of GNAT3 (the taste receptor specific G protein, GαGustducin) in a variety of human tissues, including the heart.

We previously investigated the factors contributing to cardiac TAS2R gene expression in silico (Foster et al., 2015a). Similar to rodent Tas2rs, there was no evidence of enrichment for particular transcription factor binding sites in the proximal promoter regions of the human TAS2R genes. However, we observed thatTAS2R14 (the most abundantly expressed) had the strongest evidence of regulatory activity in its promoter region, i.e., active methylation marks overlapping with the DNase I hypersensitivity cluster. On this basis, although we cannot rule out the presence of specific transcription factors that regulate

TAS2R gene expression, we reason that the proximal regulatory regions for some, but not all, TAS2R genes might show a basal level of transcriptional activity. This, combined with their multigene cluster expression profiles could facilitate preferential transcription of the specific TAS2Rs (Foster et al., 2015a).

The heart is made up of 2–3 billion cardiomyocytes and yet these cells constitute less than a third of all heart tissue (Tirziu et al., 2010). The remaining, more than two thirds of the heart consists of smooth muscle, fibroblasts, other connective tissue cells, endothelial cells, sinoatrial cells, atrioventricular cells, Purkinje cells, pluripotent cardiac stem cells, mast cells, and other immune system-related cells (Tirziu et al., 2010). We have demonstrated that certain Tas2rs (rodent) were expressed within both cardiomyocytes and fibroblasts, as well as their downstream signaling effectors (Gnat3, Plcβ2, Trpm5) (Foster et al., 2013). These data suggest that specific cells within the heart may express varying populations of TAS2R, similar to that seen in other systems (Table 1). As technology advances, including single cell sequencing and proteomics (Uhlen et al., 2015), the topography of T2Rs within the heart will provide insight into how these receptors function within this system.

Go to:

Signaling and Function of T2Rs Within the Cardiovascular System
The binding of bitter ligands to T2Rs results in a conformation change in the receptor allowing it to interact with GαGustducin and Gβ1/3γ13 (Huang et al., 1999), which then activate subsequent downstream pathways (Yan et al., 2001). Knockout (KO) studies have provided conclusive evidence supporting these signaling pathways. Mice lacking either PLCβ2 or TRPM5 exhibited diminished or ablated taste responses to bitter compounds (Zhang et al., 2003). Furthermore, GαGustducin KO mice had increased levels of cAMP, compared to the wild-type mice as well as displaying severely impaired responses to the tested compounds (Clapp et al., 2008). As with Gαi-family G proteins, GαGustducin can decrease the levels of cAMP, via the activation of phosphodiesterases, which has been

observed in response to two bitter compounds, denatonium and strychnine (Yan et al., 2001). Finally, mice that were genetically modified to express novel human T2Rs demonstrated a strong aversive response to ligands that was not evident in wild-type mice (Mueller et al., 2005).

With the discovery of TAS2R expression in cardiac tissue (Foster et al., 2013), defining the signaling transduction pathway is of particular interest, yet there is limited evidence for the presence of all the classical taste signaling components in heart. The expression of GαGustducin has been shown in human heart tissue, and is particularly enriched in cardiomyocytes (BioGPS Human Cell Type and Tissue Gene Expression Profiles RNA-seq datasets). However, studies have not observed Gγ13 (Huang et al., 1999) or TRPM5 (Demir et al., 2014). TRPM4 is present within human heart tissues (Guinamard et al., 2004; Demir et al., 2014), however, both TRPM4 and TRMP5 are considered necessary for taste signal transduction (Dutta Banik et al., 2018). Hence, alternative signal transduction pathways that could mediate the effects of taste receptors in the cardiovascular system should be considered.

A study by Ueda et al. (2003) demonstrated that T2R16 could couple to a chimeric G protein consisting of the N-terminus of Gα16 and the last 44 amino acids of either GαGustducin, Gαt2or Gαi2. Furthermore, the expression of all three of these Gα subunits have been identified in taste receptor cells, with the frequency of Gαi2 being higher than that of GαGustducin (Ueda et al., 2003). Figure 1 shows a comparison of GαGustducin and Gαi2, highlighting the highly conserved amino acid residues and the region known to interact with TAS2Rs. Substitution of glycine352 for proline in GαGustducin disrupts T2R interaction with GαGustducin, although its coupling to the Gβγ and effector molecules was preserved (Ruiz-Avila et al., 2001). This suggests that the extreme C terminus of both GαGustducin and Gαi2 are capable of, and necessary for T2R:G protein coupling and transduction. Importantly, in human airway smooth muscle (HASM), the reported expression of Gαi2 expression was 100-fold higher than that of GαGustducin and T2R14 was shown to couple to all Gαi proteins, particularly Gαi2 (Kim et al., 2017). The use of pertussis toxin was able to abrogate the T2R mediated relaxation in HASM (Kim et al., 2017), consistent with previous studies, where T2Rs has been shown to couple with inhibitory signaling pathways (Ozeck et al., 2004). The actions of T2R may also include other inhibitory type processes, such as described by Zhang et al. (2013) in airway smooth muscle cells (Lu et al., 2017). Taken together these observations suggest that depending on the level of G protein expression and the strength of the subsequent signal, T2Rs likely couple and signal in a cell/tissue specific manner, which may include (or not) GαGustducin.

Comparison of 2D snake representations of GαGustducin and Gαi2 [constructed via GPCRdb (Isberg et al., 2016)]. Amino acids are labeled following the Ballesteros–Weinstein numbering system. Conserved amino acids are colored green. The final 44 amino acids are known to be necessary for T2R coupling and signaling (Ueda et al., 2003) and are highlighted by black boxes. Arrow points to the amino acid (Glycine352) in GαGustducin that disrupts T2R coupling when mutated to proline (Ruiz-Avila et al., 2001).

Indeed, T2R signaling within cardiac cells might reasonably reflect those described for the respiratory system and vascular systems (summarized in Figure 2). The heart is known to express specific varying combinations of Gα (including Gαi2), Gβγ and various signaling effector molecules (Doll et al., 2017). In a series of experiments in Langendorff-perfused mouse hearts, we observed dose-dependent negative inotropic effects in response to bitter ligands (Foster et al., 2014). A ~40% decrease in left ventricular developed pressure and an increase in aortic pressure in response to sodium thiocynate were shown to be Gαi-dependent. Some alterations in cardiovascular physiology were not attributed to G proteins (not blocked by pertussis toxin and gallein), however, it was shown that rodents express

GNAT3 (GαGustducin) in their cardiomyocytes (Foster et al., 2013). This further supports the premise that T2Rs can signal through various G proteins. While there is no clear consensus on the precise mechanism, there is an agreement that bitter ligands mediate contractile responses in the vasculature. One study demonstrated a transient drop in blood pressure upon intravenous injection of denatonium benzoate into rats (Lund et al., 2013). Additionally, Manson et al. (2014) attributed the endothelium-independent relaxation of precontracted human pulmonary arteries to the application of bitter ligands for T2Rs (3, 4, 10, and 14). In contrast, denatonium benzoate has been shown to enhance the tone of endothelium-denuded rat aorta rings, which was attributed to specific Tas2r activation (Tas2r40, 108, 126, 135, 137, 143) via GαGustducin (Liu et al., 2020). Whether the actions of T2Rs in cardiomyocytes have a direct effect on the force and strength of contraction of individual myocytes remains to be determined. Equally, there is a possibility that these receptors may be expressed in other cell populations, including the specific cells of the conduction system (SA node, AV node, Purkinje Fibers).

Potential signaling pathway for T2Rs in human cardiomyocytes.
Go to:
Naturally Occurring Polymorphisms and Disease
GPCRs and their respective ligands have profound homeostatic and regulatory effects on the cardiovascular system. Not surprisingly, mutations and modifications of cardiovascular GPCRs, G proteins and their regulatory proteins are linked to dysfunction and disease (Foster et al., 2015b). T2Rs are one of the most heterogenous and unique families of GPCRs and are now considered as a separate group of receptors (Di Pizio and Niv, 2015). According to the HGNC database, there are 39 genetically diverse and highly polymorphic TAS2R single exon genes that encode for 29 functional T2Rs (and 10 non-coding pseudogenes) in humans (Devillier et al., 2015). This is in

contrast to the majority of literature that cite the existence of only 25 functional T2Rs (Meyerhof et al., 2010; Lossow et al., 2016). On average, TAS2R genes contain four single nucleotide polymorphisms (SNPs) of which the vast majority are non-synonyms mutations that encode amino acid substitutions (Kim et al., 2005). Table 2 outlines all of the non-synonymous SNPs present within the population and their penetrance. These TAS2R genes are located on chromosomes 5, 7, and 12 (Adler et al., 2000; Foster et al., 2015a), with dense clustering on chromosomes 7 and 12. The close proximity is thought to underpin the enormous variation and diversification of the T2R repertoire within humans.

TABLE 2

List of polymorphisms in human cardiac-expressed TAS2Rs (penetrance > 1% in the population) sourced from UCSC Genome Browser and NCBI SNP databases.

Open in a separate window

Italicized polymorphisms represent those that have less than 300 alleles detected in the sample population (* denotes stop codon).

The importance of uncovering the primary function of T2Rs in the heart is supported by the critical role they play within the respiratory system. TAS2R38 is expressed in all aspects of the upper and lower respiratory tracts including sinonasal epithelial cells, bronchial epithelial cells, bronchial smooth muscle, and pulmonary vasculature smooth muscle (Shah et al., 2009; Grassin-Delyle et al., 2013; Upadhyaya et al., 2014; Devillier et al., 2015). Application of phenylthiocarbamide (PTC) or two quorum sensing molecules (C4HSL and C12HSL) secreted by Pseudomonas aeruginosa were shown to increase mucociliary clearance, bronchodilation, and production of bactericidal levels nitric oxide in explanted human tissue samples and primary airway–liquid interface cultures (Lee et al., 2012). This supports the recent finding that T2Rs play a role in innate immunity, as quorum sensing molecules serve to communicate between bacterial populations, allowing them to establish themselves during infection (Lee et al., 2014). Bitter taste receptors, particularly TAS2R38, are a unique and diverse family of GPCRs due to the number of their naturally occurring genetic variants (Kim et al., 2005). Compared to the functional (PAV) haplotype, individuals with the non-functional (AVI) haplotype were shown to be more susceptible to respiratory infections as the receptor was unable to detect the compounds and respond appropriately (Lee et al., 2012). A similar result was seen with regard to oral innate immunity (Gil et al., 2015). TAS2R38 PAV/PAV mRNA was upregulated ~ 4.3-fold in response to Streptococcus mutans bacteria (over the unstimulated control) whereas the AVI/AVI was only ~ 1.2-fold. Furthermore, the level of hBD-2 (antimicrobial peptide) induced was highest in those with the PAV/PAV genotype (Gil et al., 2015). On this basis, the authors concluded that a person's T2R38 genotype determines oral innate immunity.

Natural polymorphisms are no longer thought only to account for differences in oral bitter taste perception (Roudnitzky et al., 2016). It is now recognized that these polymorphisms also influence other important aspects of our physiology including alcohol dependence, eating behavior, longevity, glucose homeostasis and regulation of thyroid hormones (Dotson, 2008; Hayes et al., 2011; Campa et al., 2012; Clark et al., 2015). There are 132 naturally occurring non-synonymous polymorphisms for cardiac-expressed T2Rs and it is clear that the majority of these remain uncharacterized (Table 3). One polymorphism that is of particular interest is T2R50-rs1376251, as debate remains in the literature over its potential association with myocardial infarction and coronary heart disease (Shiffman et al., 2008; Tepper et al., 2008; Yan et al., 2009; Koch et al., 2011; Ivanova et al., 2017; Tsygankova et al., 2017). There are also polymorphisms outside of the taste receptor coding region, or those that result in synonymous mutations that have been associated with changes in physiology. Of note, T2R14 rs3741843 has been associated with decreased sperm motility (Gentiluomo et al., 2017). Individuals that were homozygous carriers for the

(G) allele, encoding arginine (R – AGG), showed a decreased sperm progressive motility compared to heterozygotes and homozygotes for the (A) allele, which encodes arginine (R – AGA). The authors rationalized using in silico analysis that T2R14 regulates the expression of T2R43. Furthermore, an upstream mutation of TAS2R3 rs11763979 can regulate the expression of WEE2 antisense RNA one (WEE2-AS1), which increases the expression of WEE2 within the testis. WEE2 is a protein tyrosine kinase involved in the regulation of cell cycle progression (Nakanishi et al., 2000). Overexpression of WEE2 in the testis was hypothesized to increase the number of abnormal sperm cells (Gentiluomo et al., 2017). Despite recent progress, it is unclear the full extent to which polymorphisms can influence T2R physiology, although it is clear investigation into their effects is warranted.

TABLE 3

List of ligands known to activate cardiac specific T2Rs and their classification, number of T2Rs activated [bold indicates the receptor corresponding to the lowest threshold (TC) or effective concentration (EC50) in vitro concentration], reported effects in the cardiovascular system and corresponding dose/serum (* = based on 5.5 L of blood in human body, or without First Pass Effect of liver).

Open in a separate window
Go to:
Potential Cardiovascular T2R Ligands
T2Rs are unique as they lack most of the conserved motifs of the class A GPCR family (Lagerstrom and Schioth, 2008). The intracellular loops – regions necessary for signal transduction and feedback modulation (Moreira, 2014), were shown to be more conserved across T2Rs than the extracellular loops that are generally implicated in receptor binding (Meyerhof, 2005). Using T2R14 as an example, Nowak et al. (2018) demonstrated that in vitro mutagenesis of 19 receptor mutants (all within the binding pocket) retained the ability to bind at least one of the 7 tested agonists while some improved signaling compared to the

wild type. These results are consistent with previous literature that ligands bind within the transmembrane and extracellular domain regions (Brockhoff et al., 2010; Upadhyaya et al., 2015). Interestingly, of the highly expressed cardiac T2Rs, T2R10, T2R14, and T2R46 were shown to bind a wide array of ligands, which is considered disproportional in comparison to the others (Meyerhof et al., 2010). Over 75% of the list of ligands in Table 3 were shown to activate these three broadly tuned T2Rs.

Universally, researchers have used chemicals that 'taste bitter 'to test for potential ligands. However, if heart tissue expresses over half of the T2Rs family, a major question arises - what is the source of ligands for these T2Rs within the cardiovascular system? We would argue there are four major sources: (1) bitter compounds in food, (2) endogenously produced factors, (3) bacterial metabolic by-products and toxins and (4) chemicals/drugs (outlined in Table 3).

The post-prandial concentration of bitter compounds in the blood increases. One perhaps common example of this is caffeine, which reportedly modulates calcium signaling via interaction with the ryanodine receptor (Kong et al., 2008). Interestingly, caffeine also activates T2R10, -14, and -46 (Meyerhof et al., 2010; Cappelletti et al., 2018) at concentrations that occur in blood post-prandially and which are equivalent to levels that modulate the ryanodine receptor (Kong et al., 2008). In the gut, caffeine activation of T2R has been linked to gastric secretion (Liszt et al., 2017). Caffeine may also act as a stimulate for the central nervous system via the antagonism of adenosine receptors (Fisone et al., 2004). Hence in considering the homeostatic consequence of bitter compounds (such as caffeine) one must also accept that at high concentrations they are interacting with multiple receptor systems. We would anticipate that many bitter compounds in food would have actions on both T2Rs and other targets.

Another interesting possibility is that the body produces endogenous factors that could activate T2Rs. Currently, alanine, pantothenic acid (vitamin B5), steroids (androsterone and progesterone) and taurocholic acid (primary bile acid) have all been identified as ligands for specific receptors (Ji et al., 2014; Lossow et al., 2016). Potentially, the cardiotonic steroids may be ligands for cardiac-expressed T2Rs, although ouabain has already been shown not to be an agonist in vitro (Meyerhof et al., 2010), despite being able to augment calcium transients in arterial smooth muscle (Arnon et al., 2000). The other members of this family could also be investigated as potential ligands for cardiac T2Rs. Whether hormones/factors produced by other tissues, or indeed paracrine factors released from cardiac cells, can bind and activate cardiac T2Rs remains to be determined, but is an area of intense interest.

A more provocative idea is that colonizing bacteria, in complex organisms, could produce bitter compounds, including metabolic by-products and other signaling molecules that alter our physiology via T2Rs. A recent study showed commensal bacteria are enable to synthesize GPCR ligands that mimic human signaling molecules (Cohen et al., 2017). Broad screening for bacterial metabolites that activate GPCRs (Chen et al., 2019; Colosimo et al., 2019) have identified numerous candidates, but unfortunately these screens have not included the taste receptors. Interestingly, an olfactory receptor (Olfr78) has been reported to respond to short chain fatty acids produced by gut bacteria (Pluznick et al., 2013). Olfr78 KO mice had elevated blood pressure when treated with antibiotics. As for the T2Rs, T2R38 although its expression is low in the heart, was shown to be broadly tuned for seven bacterial metabolites (Verbeurgt et al., 2017). It is also worth noting that during infections bacterial toxins could be 'bitter 'and interact with T2Rs once they reached a certain concentration in the blood. One example is quorum sensing molecules - when they reach a certain concentration, bacteria produce a biofilm in order to evade and survive the host immune defense system (Davies et al., 1998). Therefore, it is plausible that T2Rs may alter cardiovascular physiology in response to systemic infections such as sepsis where dramatic cardiovascular changes are observed, e.g., decreased myocardial contractility, vasodilation, endothelial injury and increased heart rate (Singer et al., 2016).

Finally, it is important to address the possibility that off-target activation of T2Rs may play a role beyond normal physiology and mediate unexpected responses to therapeutic drugs, many of which are bitter. Indeed, the possibility that T2Rs act as the mediators of off-target drug effects due to the prevalence of their expression throughout the body has been discussed previously (Clark et al., 2012). There are numerous drugs/chemicals that have specific, detrimental cardiovascular effects and, moreover, these chemicals have been shown to activate specific T2Rs at concentrations to those that elicit these adverse effects.

Future Directions

The continuous, proper functioning of the heart is fundamental to life. The discovery of T2Rs expressed in cardiac cells predicts important (but yet to be appreciated) roles in heart physiology, as well as its response to external challenges (e.g., diet, metabolic changes, infections, and drugs). Research and knowledge regarding the physiology of T2Rs within the human heart is challenging, primarily due to the constraints of readily acquiring suitable human heart tissue samples. Furthermore, the lack of homology between rodent Tas2rs and human T2Rs (Foster et al., 2013), limits the utility of gene modified animal models to directly inform human physiology. Additionally, the 29 T2Rs (and their many variants) have been historically difficult to heterologously express on the cell membrane of model cells, and this has impeded further investigation of their signaling properties.

It is important to note, that researchers have ectopically expressed human T2Rs in mice and this has provided strong confirmation that a given ligand (tastants) can activate a specific human T2R (Mueller et al., 2005). Perhaps future experiments might extend this approach to develop transgenic mice expressing human T2Rs in a cell-specific context. Stimulation of these receptors with ligands that selectively bind and activate only human T2Rs could provide important insights into the physiological role(s) of T2Rs in human tissues.

Another critical objective will be to develop appropriate cardiac models that express endogenous receptors and recapitulate cardiac physiology. One major advance in cardiovascular research has been the development of induced pluripotent stem cell-derived human cardiomyocytes (Hudson et al., 2012; Soong et al., 2012) and human cardiac organoids (Nugraha et al., 2019). These models will offer the unique opportunity to modulate T2R expression in cardiomyocytes and to thereby investigate bitter ligand-driven changes in cardiac gene transcription, as well as to define alterations in cardiac contractility and function.

Finally, the ultimate goal will be to attribute T2R-mediated expression, activation and signaling to definitive changes in human cardiovascular function in vivo. In order for this to succeed, the following challenges need to be resolved - the promiscuity of bitter receptor–ligand interactions, the elucidation of tissue-specific T2R signaling, as well as the lack of definitive research tools (e.g., selective antibodies to T2Rs and specific receptor antagonists). We anticipate that studies focused on examining the functionality (or lack thereof) for the various highly penetrant, cardiac-expressed T2R polymorphisms may provide the means for unambiguously attributing T2R activation to a specific physiological outcome. Analogous to the advances made with non-functional T2R38 variants (T2R38AVI) in the lung, we predict that non-functional, cardiac-expressed T2Rs can be identified and these will prove to be critical in providing the necessary controls for investigating explanted cardiac tissues.

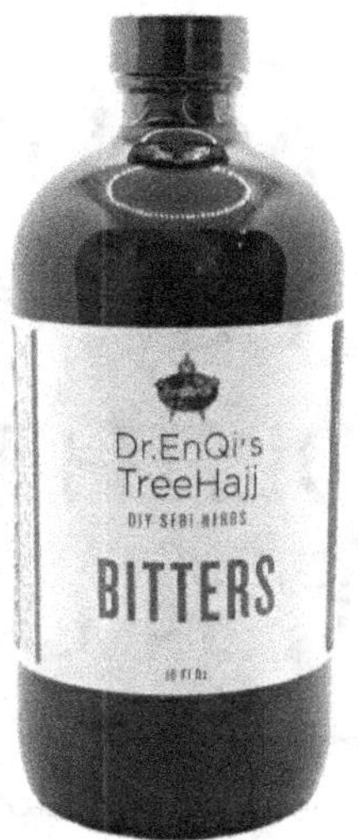

AMERICANHEALER.WEBSITE

PHARMACOLOGICAL EFFECTS OF UROLITHIN A AND ITS ROLE IN MUSCLE HEALTH AND PERFORMANCE: CURRENT KNOWLEDGE AND PROSPECTS

Haotian Zhao,1,2,† Ge Song,3,† Hongkang Zhu,2,† He Qian,2 Xinliang Pan,3 Xiaoneng Song,1,* Yijie Xie,4,* and Chang Liu3,*
David C. Nieman, Academic Editor and John.A. Rathmacher, Academic Editor
Author information Article notes Copyright and License information PMC Disclaimer

Abstract

Urolithin A (UA) is a naturally occurring compound derived from the metabolism of gut microbiota, which has attracted considerable research attention due to its pharmacological effects and potential implications in muscle health and performance. Recent studies have demonstrated that Urolithin A exhibits diverse biological activities, encompassing anti-inflammatory, antioxidant, anti-tumor, and anti-aging properties. In terms of muscle health, accumulating evidence suggests that Urolithin A may promote muscle protein synthesis and muscle growth through various pathways, offering promise in mitigating muscle atrophy. Moreover, Urolithin A exhibits the potential to enhance muscle health and performance by improving mitochondrial function and regulating autophagy. Nonetheless, further comprehensive investigations are still warranted to elucidate the underlying mechanisms of Urolithin A and to assess its feasibility and safety in human subjects, thereby advancing its potential applications in the realms of muscle health and performance.

Keywords: Urolithin A, muscle health, muscle performance, pharmacology, review

1. Introduction

In recent years, there has been a substantial increase in the recognition of the critical importance of both health and athletic performance [1,2]. The pursuit of muscle health and optimal athletic performance is no longer confined solely to athletes or fitness enthusiasts but has become a pervasive goal among the general population, who strive for a healthier and more active lifestyle [3,4]. Consequently, there is a widespread demand for strategies to enhance muscle health and improve athletic performance, rendering this field an area of profound discussion and extensive research.

Urolithin A, a naturally occurring compound derived from dietary sources, has swiftly emerged as a prominent subject of investigation in the context of muscle health and performance [5,6,7]. Existing evidence supports the potential of Urolithin A in facilitating muscle cell proliferation and augmenting muscle function (Figure 1) [8,9,10]. However, the understanding of the mechanisms of action and potential applications of Urolithin A as it relates to muscle health and athletic performance is still in its infancy.

Pharmacological effects of Urolithin A and its role in promoting muscle health and enhancing athletic performance.

The present review aims to provide a comprehensive survey and analysis of current research on the impact of Urolithin A on muscle health and performance, as well as suggest directions for future research. The topic will be examined from multiple perspectives, consolidating and assessing existing experimental outcomes to unravel the correlation between Urolithin A, muscle health, and corresponding biological processes and molecular mechanisms. Furthermore, potential areas of application of Urolithin A, including its feasibility as a dietary supplement or pharmaceutical product, will be discussed. This paper, grounded in an extensive literature review and systematic analysis, seeks to synthesize current research findings to offer fresh insights into the role of Urolithin A in muscle health and performance. It is anticipated that these insights may provide valuable guidance for further exploration into the functional mechanisms of Urolithin A, ultimately facilitating the development of innovative strategies to enhance muscle health.

2. Urolithin A's Sources in the Diet

Urolithin A, a natural metabolite derived from ellagitannins, is biosynthesized by the gut microbiota [11,12], It is a type of compound known as urolithins, which are present in pomegranates and certain other fruits and nuts such as strawberries, walnut kernels, and peanuts. Ellagitannins serve as precursors to urolithins and undergo microbial metabolism within the gastrointestinal tract to produce Urolithin A [7]. Pomegranate, walnut, and almond stand out as the primary and richest dietary sources of Urolithin A [13,14]. Pomegranate peel and seeds contain abundant polyphenolic compounds, including Urolithin A formed through metabolism by the gut microbiota. Walnut is also considered a dietary source of Urolithin A, as it is rich in polyphenolic compounds and anthocyanins that may interact with gut microbiota during digestion and potentially generate Urolithin A. Almond is another potential dietary source of Urolithin A. It contains polyphenolic compounds, particularly flavonoids and anthocyanins, which can be converted into Urolithin A upon interaction with gut microbiota. Blueberry, recognized for its antioxidant-rich content, including various polyphenolic compounds, which may also include Urolithin A [15]. However, research on the content of Urolithin A in blueberry remains limited, necessitating further studies to confirm its source and concentration [16].

3. Metabolism and Bioavailability of Urolithin A in the Body

3.1. Gut Microbiota Metabolism

The production of Urolithin A is largely dependent on the metabolic activities of gut microbiota [7]. During the process of digestion, several polyphenolic compounds found in food such as tannins and anthocyanins, undergo enzymatic reactions and metabolic conversions facilitated by microbial enzymes, culminating in the production of Urolithin A [17]. This metabolism predominantly takes place in the colon, which houses a variety of microbial groups. These groups, including Proteobacteria, Clostridium, Bifidobacterium, Eubacterium, and Enterococcus faecium possess distinct metabolic functions that play a part in the production of Urolithin A (Figure 2) [18,19,20,21,22].

The metabolism, bioavailability, pharmacological effects, and impact on muscle health of Urolithin A.

3.2. Absorption, Distribution, Metabolism, and Excretion

Following absorption in the intestines, Urolithin A enters the circulatory system and is transported to various tissues and organs through the bloodstream [11,23]. Studies have indicated that in the human body, Urolithin A primarily exists in a free form rather than being bound to other molecules [24]. Once inside the cell, Urolithin A undergoes further metabolism through multiple metabolic pathways [25]. One prominent pathway involves the conversion of Urolithin A into its mercaptan and sulfate forms, facilitated by metabolic enzymes present in the liver [26]. Furthermore, some studies have suggested that Urolithin A may participate in metabolic processes such as glucose metabolism and fatty acid oxidation. Urolithin A and its metabolites can be excreted from the body through the kidneys and intestines [25]. A portion of Urolithin A is further metabolized into other compounds within the intestines before being eliminated through feces [24]. These processes may be influenced by factors such as intestinal permeability, renal function, and individual characteristics.

It is important to note that the metabolism and utilization of Urolithin A may vary among individuals, depending on their intestinal microbial composition, metabolic capacity, genetic factors, dietary habits, and other physiological states [8,27]. Furthermore, the bioavailability of Urolithin A may also be influenced by the dietary source, intake level, and tissue specificity [28]. Although some insights into the metabolic mechanisms and bioavailability of Urolithin A have been gained, further research is still needed to comprehensively understand its behavior and effects in the human body, as well as its associations with relevant health effects.

3.3. Factors Influencing the Absorption and Distribution of Urolithin A

3.3.1. Dietary Components

The absorption and distribution of Urolithin A can be influenced by compounds present in food. For instance, the consumption of polyphenolic-rich foods, such as pomegranate, walnuts, almonds, and others, can supply an abundance of precursor molecules for intestinal microbial metabolism, facilitating the generation of Urolithin A [29,30,31]. Moreover, certain components in food may compete with Urolithin A for absorption within the gastrointestinal tract, consequently impacting its bioavailability [24].

3.3.2. Composition and Activity of the Gut Microbiota

The composition and activity of an individual's intestinal microbiota play a pivotal role in Urolithin A metabolism and absorption [32]. The gut microbial communities in different individuals may exhibit distinct capabilities in converting polyphenolic compounds present in food into Urolithin A [33]. Therefore, interindividual variations could potentially impact the bioavailability of Urolithin A.

3.3.3. Individual Variations

Individual variations can also have an impact on the absorption and distribution of Urolithin A. Genetic factors, for instance, can lead to interindividual differences in the activity and expression of metabolic enzymes, which can affect the rate of Urolithin A metabolism. Additionally, variations in intestinal permeability, the health status of the digestive system, and other physiological states may impact the absorption and distribution of Urolithin A [34].

3.3.4. Drug Interactions

Currently, there is a lack of direct research on the effects of drugs on the metabolism and clearance processes of Urolithin A. However, certain drugs may interact with Urolithin A and affect its absorption and metabolism. For example, specific drugs may competitively inhibit or induce metabolic enzymes, interfering with the metabolism and clearance of Urolithin A. Drug interactions with cytochrome P450 (CYP450) enzymes in the liver, for instance, can competitively inhibit or induce these enzyme, thereby disrupting the metabolism and clearance of Urolithin A [35]. Commonly used antibiotics, antifungal drugs, and anticancer drugs have been reported to interact with CYP450 enzymes [36]. Hepatic enzyme inducers, such as rifampicin and carbamazepine, can increase the activity of certain metabolic enzymes in the liver, potentially accelerating the metabolism of Urolithin A and reducing its half-life in the body [37]. Certain drugs, such as clarithromycin, can inhibit the activity of metabolic enzymes in the liver, slowing down the metabolism and clearance processes of Urolithin A and leading to its accumulation in the body [38].

Although the factors mentioned above may influence the absorption and distribution of Urolithin A, further research is essential to gain a more precise understanding of their specific effects on the metabolism and bioavailability of Urolithin A. Continued studies will contribute to a more comprehensive comprehension of Urolithin A's behavior and effects, offering more accurate guidance for its application in health management.

4. Pharmacological Effects of Urolithin A

4.1. Activation of Mitochondrial Autophagy and Regeneration

Mitochondrial autophagy, also known as mitophagy, refers to the selective degradation of mitochondria through the autophagic process. This process typically occurs in mitochondria that are damaged or defective due to stress. Mitochondrial autophagy plays a pivotal role in maintaining cellular health by facilitating the turnover of mitochondria and preventing the accumulation of dysfunctional ones, which could otherwise lead to cellular degeneration. The regulation of mitochondrial autophagy is mediated by proteins such as PINK1 and Parkin [39,40,41].

Apart from its function in selectively eliminating damaged mitochondria, mitochondrial autophagy is essential for adjusting the mitochondrial population to meet changing cellular metabolic demands, ensuring mitochondrial turnover and homeostasis. Research has demonstrated that Urolithin A activates the PINK1/Parkin signaling pathway, which is involved in mitochondrial quality control. Consequently, this activation promotes the selective aggregation, degradation, and removal of damaged mitochondria [42].

Furthermore, research has illuminated Urolithin A's capacity to enhance mitochondrial autophagy by activating the expression of glutathione S-transferases (GSTs). GSTs are pivotal detoxifying enzymes intricately related to antioxidant capacity. Urolithin A stimulates the Nrf2-ARE signaling pathway, subsequently upregulating the expression of GSTs, thereby enhancing cellular autophagy and mitochondrial quality control [43].

In summary, Urolithin A participates in regulating mitochondrial autophagy and quality control by activating the PINK1/Parkin and glutathione S-transferases signaling pathway.

4.2. Antioxidant Activity

Antioxidant activity refers to the capacity to inhibit oxidation, a chemical reaction that typically involves the generation of free radicals, often through autoxidation processes. Urolithin A exhibits antioxidant activity through multiple mechanisms. Firstly, it possesses the ability to directly scavenge free radicals by capturing and neutralizing reactive oxygen species such as peroxy radicals and superoxide radicals, thus reducing cellular oxidative stress [44]. Secondly, Urolithin A can activate the Nrf2 antioxidant pathway [45] and upregulate the expression of various antioxidant enzymes such as Glutathione peroxidase and superoxide dismutase, thereby enhancing cellular antioxidant defense capacity. Additionally, Urolithin A has been reported to inhibit enzyme activities involved in ROS generation, thereby reducing the occurrence of oxidative stress and protecting cells from oxidative damage [46].

4.3. Regulation of Cell Cycle and Cell Apoptosis

Research has shown that Urolithin A can regulate the cell cycle and induce apoptosis [47]. In terms of cell cycle regulation, Urolithin A can impact cell cycle-related protein kinase complexes, such as cyclin-dependent kinases (CDKs) and cyclins. It inhibits the activity of CDKs and reduces the expression of cell cycle proteins such as cyclin D1, leading to cell cycle arrest in the G1 phase [47]. Additionally, Urolithin A can regulate the cell cycle by increasing the levels of cell cycle inhibitory proteins, such as p21 and p27 [48,49].

Regarding apoptosis, Urolithin A can induce cell death through multiple pathways. Studies have found that Urolithin A increases the Bax/Bcl-2 ratio, resulting in the loss of mitochondrial membrane potential, release of cytochrome c, and activation of caspase cascades, ultimately leading to cell apoptosis [49]. Furthermore, Urolithin A can activate the JNK (c-Jun N-terminal kinase) and p38 MAPK (mitogen-activated protein kinase) signaling pathways, further promoting apoptosis [50].

4.4. Influences on Metabolic Regulation

Urolithin A participates in the regulation of multiple metabolic pathways. Research has shown that Urolithin A can activate the adenosine monophosphate-activated protein kinase (AMPK) signaling pathway, which is a pivotal regulator of energy metabolism [51]. Activation of AMPK promotes fatty acid oxidation and insulin sensitivity while reducing fatty acid synthesis and gluconeogenesis [51,52]. Additionally, Urolithin A can modulate the activity of peroxisome proliferator-activated receptor gamma (PPARγ) [53], a crucial transcription factor involved in adipocyte differentiation, glucose metabolism, and cholesterol metabolism, among other processes [54]. Studies have indicated that Urolithin A can increase the expression of PPARγ and transcription of its downstream target genes, thereby promoting fatty acid oxidation, improving insulin sensitivity, and reducing cholesterol synthesis and absorption [53].

In conclusion, Urolithin A regulates the cell cycle by activating the Nrf2 and PINK1/Parkin signaling pathways, inhibiting ROS production, and modulating the activity of CDKs and cyclins. It also induces cell apoptosis through the modulation of the Bax/Bcl-2 ratio and activation of the JNK/p38 MAPK signaling pathways. Additionally, Urolithin A's regulatory effects involve the activation of metabolic regulators such as AMPK and PPARγ. These molecular mechanisms collectively contribute to the various cellular and biological effects of Urolithin A. Further research is needed to unravel the detailed mechanisms of Urolithin A and its interactions with other signaling pathways.

5. The Effects of Urolithin A on Muscle Health

5.1. The Antioxidant Activity of Urolithin A

Oxidative stress results from an excess production of free radicals and reactive oxygen species (ROS) [55]. During exercise, especially strenuous activities, the body is more susceptible to generating an excessive amount of ROS, and these reactive substances can inflict damage on cellular structures and functions. Urolithin A, functioning as an antioxidant, can neutralize free radicals and mitigate their harmful effects to cells. This action can lower the level of oxidative stress within muscle cells and protect cellular structures and functions, thereby promoting muscle health.

Urolithin A may also be able to activate critical antioxidant enzymes in the body, such as superoxide dismutase (SOD) and Glutathione peroxidase (GPx). These enzymes actively scavenge free radicals and peroxides within cells, reducing the extent of oxidative stress and contributing to muscle health. Additionally, Urolithin A can further promote the synthesis of certain antioxidant molecules, such as glutathione (GSH), glutathione S-transferase, etc. [44]. These molecules play a vital role in regulating oxidative stress and preserving the health of muscle cells.

Furthermore, the antioxidant properties of Urolithin A can reduce the occurrence of inflammatory reactions [56]. Oxidative stress and inflammation are often intertwined, mutually exacerbating each other. Urolithin A may attenuate the intensity of inflammatory responses by alleviating oxidative stress, thereby exerting a positive impact on muscle health.

5.2. The Anti-Inflammatory Effects of Urolithin A

Urolithin A possesses significant anti-inflammatory effects, which are instrumental for muscle recovery. During exercise and physical exertion, muscles undergo a certain degree of damage, triggering an inflammatory response [57]. Moderate inflammation constitutes a natural process of the body's repair, but excessive or prolonged inflammation may impair muscle recovery and growth. Research has indicated that Urolithin A can inhibit the inflammatory response and alleviate inflammation-induced damage [58]. It exerts these anti-inflammatory effects through multiple mechanisms, including inhibiting the release of inflammatory mediators, suppressing the activation of inflammatory signaling pathways, and reducing oxidative stress. By suppressing the inflammatory response, Urolithin A contributes to the mitigation of muscle pain and inflammation and promotes muscle repair and recovery [59]. This is particularly important for post-exercise muscle recovery as it expedites the healing process of muscle cells, reducing muscle soreness and discomfort, and improving muscle function and performance

[57].

In addition, Urolithin A is also able to promote mitochondrial function and muscle energy metabolism, which has a positive impact on muscle recovery and performance. By enhancing mitochondrial function, Urolithin A can increase energy production and muscle cells 'ability to recover, thereby accelerating the muscle recovery process. Overall, the anti-inflammatory effects of Urolithin A are crucial for muscle recovery. It not only alleviates inflammation caused by exercise but also promotes the repair and energy metabolism of muscle cells, ultimately enhancing muscle recovery ability and performance level.

5.3. The Role of Urolithin A in Promoting Mitochondrial Function and Muscle Energy Metabolism

Urolithin A plays a substantial role in promoting mitochondrial function and muscle energy metabolism [51]. Mitochondria are the principal organelles responsible for cellular energy production and are crucial for muscle cell function and performance. Research has shown that Urolithin A can enhance mitochondrial function and activity [10]. It achieves this by activating gene expression similar to PGC-1α (transcriptional coactivator peroxisome proliferator-activated receptor γ coactivator-1α), regulating the quantity and quality of mitochondria. PGC-1α is a pivotal regulatory transcription factor involved in mitochondrial biogenesis, the formation of respiratory chain complexes, and processes such as mitochondrial fission and fusion [60,61].

Urolithin A also exhibits antioxidant properties, reducing the generation of free radicals and protecting mitochondria from oxidative stress-induced damage. Excessive free radicals production and oxidative stress can damage the structure and function of mitochondria, affecting muscle energy metabolism and recovery capacity. Urolithin A clears free radicals, protects mitochondria from damage, and improves the efficiency of energy production. Furthermore, Urolithin A can promote ATP generation in muscle cells. ATP is the primary energy molecule for muscle cells and is crucial for muscle contraction and exercise performance [62]. Research has found that Urolithin A can promote the formation and enhanced function of mitochondrial respiratory chain complexes, thereby improving the synthesis rate of ATP in muscle cells [10]. By promoting mitochondrial function and muscle energy metabolism, Urolithin A has a positive impact on muscle performance and recovery. It can increase energy supply to muscle cells and improve muscle endurance and strength performance. Additionally, Urolithin A alleviates fatigue caused by exercise and promotes rapid muscle recovery.

In summary, Urolithin A assumes a vital role in muscle performance and recovery by promoting mitochondrial function and muscle energy metabolism. It enhances mitochondrial activity, reduces oxidative stress and free radical generation, and promotes ATP synthesis, thereby improving the energy supply and physical performance in muscle cells.

6. The Effects of Urolithin A on Muscle Performance

6.1. The Potential Effects of Urolithin A on Endurance and Anti-Fatigue Capacity

Limited research currently supports the potential impact of Urolithin A on endurance and anti-fatigue capacity [9,10]. Although further research is needed, existing evidence suggests that Urolithin A may have a positive role in improving endurance and delaying muscle fatigue, both of which are intricately linked to mitochondrial function [63]. Firstly, Urolithin A can increase the energy supply of muscle cells by promoting mitochondrial function and muscle energy metabolism [7]. Mitochondria are crucial components for cellular energy production, and Urolithin A can enhance mitochondrial activity and ATP synthesis rates [8]. This bears significance for sustained exercise and endurance performance, as it can delay the onset of muscle fatigue and provide prolonged energy support. Secondly, Urolithin A possesses anti-inflammatory properties which can alleviate tissue damage and muscle soreness caused by inflammatory reactions [58]. Excessive or prolonged inflammation can lead to muscle fatigue and reduced endurance. By inhibiting inflammatory responses, Urolithin A helps alleviate muscle pain and discomfort, protects muscles from inflammation-induced injuries, and consequently enhances endurance and anti-fatigue capacity. Additionally, Urolithin A can improve muscle contraction speed and exercise efficiency, which also has a positive impact on endurance and anti-fatigue capacity [8]. This enhancement is achieved by promoting mitochondrial function and regulating muscle cell energy metabolism, enhancing the efficiency and force output of muscle contractions. This means that Urolithin A has the potential to delay the onset of fatigue and improve endurance during prolonged or high-intensity exercise.

It is essential to note that there is currently limited research available regarding the effects of Urolithin A on endurance and anti-fatigue capacity, and most studies have been conducted in vitro or on animals. Therefore, more human studies are needed to validate these potential effects and determine the optimal dosage and duration. However, the current evidence suggests that Urolithin A may hold promise for enhancing endurance and anti-fatigue capacity, especially with continuous supplementation.

6.2. The Effects of Urolithin A on Muscle Hypertrophy and Maintenance of Muscle Mass

Urolithin A may have a positive impact on muscle hypertrophy and maintenance of muscle mass. It exerts its effects through multiple pathways, including promotion of muscle cell repair and growth, enhancement of mitochondrial function and energy metabolism, and regulation of protein synthesis and degradation processes [8,53]. Firstly, Urolithin A can promote muscle cell repair and growth. During exercise and training, muscles undergo damage that requires repair and growth for muscle hypertrophy to occur [64]. Urolithin A provides a better environment for muscle cell repair and growth by promoting mitochondrial function and increasing ATP synthesis [65]. This can increase the cross-sectional area of muscle fibers, muscle protein content, and muscle strength, thus promoting muscle hypertrophy. Secondly, the regulation of protein synthesis and degradation processes by Urolithin A is also crucial for muscle hypertrophy and maintenance of muscle mass. It can increase the rate of protein synthesis within muscle cells and inhibit protein degradation processes [53]. This allows muscle cells to more effectively synthesize new proteins and maintain muscle mass. Additionally, Urolithin A can improve muscle endurance and exercise performance by promoting mitochondrial function and muscle energy metabolism [66]. This may lead to longer and more intense training sessions, further promoting muscle hypertrophy and the maintenance of muscle mass.

It should be noted that current research is still limited and mostly conducted in vitro or animal experiments. More human studies are needed to validate the potential effects of Urolithin A on muscle hypertrophy and the maintenance of muscle mass and to determine the optimal dosage and duration. However, based on current evidence, Urolithin A may have a positive impact on promoting muscle hypertrophy and maintaining muscle mass, particularly when used in combination with appropriate exercise and dietary plans [67].

7. The Signaling Pathways and Mechanisms of Action of Urolithin A in Muscle

7.1. The Interaction of Urolithin A with Key Signaling Pathways Involved in Muscle Health and Performance

7.1.1. AMPK Pathway

Urolithin A has been found to activate the AMPK (adenosine monophosphate-activated protein kinase) pathway [51]. By activating AMPK, Urolithin A can increase mitochondrial biogenesis and enhance fatty acid oxidation and glycogen synthesis, ultimately improving muscle energy supply and metabolism and enhancing muscle performance (Figure 3) [68]. The literature demonstrates that Urolithin A activates AMPK through a cascade involving the activation of SIRT3 and, subsequently, LKB1 [69].

The signaling pathways and mechanisms of action of Urolithin A in muscle.

7.1.2. mTOR Pathway

The mTOR (mammalian target of rapamycin) pathway plays a key role in regulating muscle protein synthesis and cell growth [70,71,72,73]. Research has found that Urolithin A can regulate protein synthesis and growth of muscle cells by inhibiting specific regulatory factors within the mTOR signaling pathway, such as PI3K (phosphoinositide 3-kinase) and Akt (protein kinase B) [74,75]. This regulation supports muscle growth and maintains muscle quality [70]. The literature has demonstrated that Urolithin A inhibits mTOR by first inhibiting PI3K and then AKT.

7.1.3. NF-κB Pathway

The NF-κB (nuclear factor kappa-light-chain-enhancer of activated B cells) pathway is implicated in the regulation of inflammatory responses [76,77]. Urolithin A has been found to inhibit the activation of NF-κB and reduce the production of inflammatory mediators [78,79]. By inhibiting the NF-κB pathway, Urolithin A can mitigate muscle damage and pain caused by inflammatory responses, thereby promoting muscle recovery and health [44]. The literature indicates that Urolithin A blocks the NF-κB/STAT1 Axis through the inactivation of TLR3/TRIF signaling.

7.1.4. PGC-1α Pathway

PGC-1α is an important transcription coactivator that regulates mitochondrial biogenesis and cellular energy metabolism [60,61]. Research has found that Urolithin A can enhance the expression and activation of PGC-1α, leading to improved mitochondrial function and increased mitochondrial quantity [80,81,82]. This enhancement is crucial for ensuring an adequate muscle energy supply and supporting endurance performance [83]. The scientific literature provides evidence that Urolithin A activates PGC-1α through a cascade that includes the activation of SIRT3, followed by the activation of LKB1 and AMPK.

7.2. The Regulatory Effects of Urolithin A on Muscle Protein Synthesis and Degradation

7.2.1. FoxO Family

The FoxO (forkhead box O) family is a group of transcription factors that are involved in regulating the synthesis and degradation of muscle proteins [84,85]. Studies have found that Urolithin A can inhibit the degradation of muscle proteins by suppressing the activation of FoxO [86]. This is primarily achieved by inhibiting the nuclear activity of FoxO and reducing their regulation of specific protein degradation pathways.

7.2.2. Ubiquitin-Proteasome System

The ubiquitin-proteasome system stands as one of the main pathways responsible for the degradation of intracellular proteins [87,88,89]. Studies have found that Urolithin A can attenuate the degradation of muscle proteins by inhibiting the activity of the ubiquitin–proteasome system [90]. This inhibition may be achieved by influencing the activity of specific ubiquitin ligases or proteasomes.

7.2.3. mTORC1 and Atrogin-1/MuRF1

mTORC1 (mammalian target of rapamycin complex 1) and Atrogin-1/MuRF1 (muscle-specific RING finger protein 1 and 2) are pivotal molecules involved in muscle protein synthesis and degradation [91,92,93,94]. Studies have shown that Urolithin A can regulate muscle protein synthesis and degradation by inhibiting the activity of mTORC1 [75,95] and the expression of Atrogin-1/MuRF1 [23].

8. Clinical Research Limitations and Future Perspectives

Overall, there is limited research available on the effects of Urolithin A in both physiological conditions and muscular pathologies. Key findings from existing studies are summarized below:

Effects of Urolithin A in Physiological Conditions:

1. Enhanced Muscle Function: Urolithin A has demonstrated the ability to improve muscle function in individuals with normal muscle health. It achieves this by promoting mitochondrial biogenesis, which enhances the energy production capacity of muscle cells. This enhancement results in improved muscle endurance, strength, and overall performance during physical activities [39,40,42].

2. Delaying Muscle Fatigue: Urolithin A shows promise in delaying the onset of muscle fatigue during prolonged or high-intensity exercise. By enhancing mitochondrial function and energy metabolism in muscle cells, it provides sustained energy support, enabling individuals to engage in longer and more intense training sessions [9,10,39,40,41,42].

3. Muscle Protein Synthesis: Urolithin A can stimulate muscle protein synthesis, contributing to muscle growth and maintenance. This effect is particularly beneficial for individuals looking to build and preserve muscle mass, such as athletes and fitness enthusiasts [8,53].

4. Antioxidant Defense: Urolithin A exhibits potent antioxidant properties, safeguarding muscle cells from oxidative stress and damage induced by free radicals and reactive oxygen species. This antioxidant defense is crucial for maintaining muscle health and function under normal conditions [44,45,46].

Effects of Urolithin A in Pathologies of the Muscular System:

1. Muscle Atrophy: In pathological conditions characterized by muscle atrophy, such as certain neuromuscular diseases or extended periods of immobility, Urolithin A may offer potential benefits [42,47]. It can stimulate muscle protein synthesis while inhibiting protein degradation pathways, helping to preserve muscle mass and mitigate muscle wasting [48,49].

2. Mitochondrial Dysfunction: Some muscular pathologies involve mitochondrial dysfunction, leading to reduced energy production and muscle weakness [51]. Urolithin A's capacity to enhance mitochondrial function and biogenesis holds promise in alleviating these issues, thereby improving muscle energy supply and overall function [39,40,42].

3. Inflammatory Conditions: Muscular pathologies often involve inflammation, which can exacerbate muscle damage and hinder recovery [57]. Urolithin A's anti-inflammatory properties can be valuable in reducing the intensity of inflammatory responses, promoting muscle recovery, and enhancing overall muscle health in conditions characterized by chronic inflammation [58,59].

4. Oxidative Stress: Muscular pathologies can result in increased

oxidative stress within muscle cells. Urolithin A's antioxidant activity helps mitigate oxidative damage, protecting muscle tissue and supporting its recovery and regeneration [10,44,45,46,62].

While the precise mechanisms and efficacy of Urolithin A in specific muscular pathologies require further research, its potential benefits in both physiological conditions and certain pathological states make it a compelling subject for future investigations and potential clinical applications.

Currently, most clinical studies related to Urolithin A are still in their early stages, characterized by relatively small sample sizes. Due to these limitations in study size, further research is required to confirm the reliability and widespread applicability of the results. Additionally, most studies have relatively short periods, and the long-term effects and safety of Urolithin A usage have not been adequately evaluated. Conducting long-term follow-up studies will provide insights into the long-term effects and potential risks of using Urolithin A. Furthermore, it is not yet clear what the optimal dosage and timing of Urolithin A should be. Different studies have used varying doses and regimens, making it challenging to compare and infer the most effective usage. Further research is needed to determine the optimal dosage and ideal administration strategy.

Additionally, the bioavailability and metabolism mechanisms of Urolithin A require further in-depth research. Investigating its absorption, distribution, and metabolic pathways within the body will facilitate better guidance on its use and effects. Moreover, there may be individual differences and heterogeneity in the human response to Urolithin A. Therefore, research needs to consider factors such as diet, genetics, and the environment that may interfere with and influence the effects of Urolithin A, to more accurately assess its mechanisms of action and effects. There are already some commercially available products related to Urolithin A on the market. However, the quality and purity of these products may vary, so it is important to ensure the acquisition of high-quality products from reliable sources and exercise appropriate dosage control.

In summary, although Urolithin A exhibits promising potential and positive effects, current research still faces challenges and limitations. Future studies need to address these issues and conduct larger-scale, long-term follow-up clinical studies to further validate the mechanisms of action, dosage effects, and safety of Urolithin A.

9. Future Research Directions and Potential Applications of Urolithin A in Exercise Science

Further long-term follow-up studies are imperative to gain a comprehensive understanding of the effects of prolonged use of Urolithin A on muscle health, exercise performance, and recovery. These studies can assess the long-term safety, efficacy, and enduring impact of Urolithin A on muscle function and recovery. Additionally, expanding the scale of research and conducting larger clinical trials will aid in confirming the effects of Urolithin A. This will aid in determining the optimal dosage, timing, and duration of Urolithin A usage, as well as evaluating its applicability to different populations and types of exercise. Further research is still required to investigate the mechanisms of action of Urolithin A in critical biological processes such as muscle metabolism, mitochondrial function, and protein synthesis/ degradation. Through these studies, a better understanding of the interaction between Urolithin A and crucial signaling pathways, as well as how it regulates muscle biological processes, can provide more mechanistic explanations for its application in exercise.

Research exploring the effects of Urolithin A in different populations such as the elderly, athletes, and individuals with muscle injuries or diseases can determine the applicability of Urolithin A in specific populations and understand its potential benefits and safety in these populations. Studies conducting exploratory studies on the interactions of Urolithin A with other nutrients (such as proteins, amino acids, etc.) or medications can evaluate the synergistic effects of Urolithin A with other interventions and determine the optimal combination strategies to enhance muscle health and exercise performance. Additionally, exploring the impact of Urolithin A on muscle gene regulation through gene expression analysis and genetic studies can elucidate the molecular mechanisms of Urolithin A in muscle health and exercise adaptation, providing valuable information for personalized exercise interventions.

In conclusion, future research should continue to delve deeper into the potential applications of Urolithin A in sports and exercise science. These endeavors will further validate its mechanisms of action, dosage effects, and safety considerations while taking into account the applicability to different populations and individual variances. Such studies will contribute to providing more specific and reliable guidance for the use of Urolithin A in sports.

10. Conclusions

In conclusion, key findings regarding Urolithin A in muscle health and performance encompass its regulatory effects on promoting muscle protein synthesis while inhibiting degradation, its interactions with crucial signaling pathways, potential enhancement of endurance and fatigue resistance, as well as its anti-inflammatory properties. These findings establish a solid scientific foundation for the potential application of Urolithin A in improving muscle health, promoting muscle growth, and enhancing exercise performance. However, further research is needed to validate these findings and to explore the safety, optimal usage, and suitable populations for Urolithin A.

MUSCLE DIGESTION WORK POST MEAL

Toe Raises alternate with Heel Raises
Sissy Squats alternate with Regular Squats
Couple Sets none stop 3-5 minutes…
Great for Circulation

Of course this can be coupled with or be replaced by a walk or any other skeletal muscle work you would prefer… The legs should become a primary focus for clearing the blood via "Complete Digestion"…

1 OR 2 SETS OF FEET, CALF, UPPER LEG AND PUSHUPS OR PULL UPS… 3-5 MINUTES FULL BODY WORK GREAT FOR DIGESTION!!! LETS START USING EXERCISE FOR DIGESTION AND BITTERS FOR CARDIO!!!